One Hundred Years of the National Formulary

One Hundred Years of the National Formulary:
A Symposium

Gregory J. Higby, Editor

Presented at a special session of the 1988 AIHP Annual Meeting, co-sponsored by the American Institute of the History of Pharmacy and the United States Pharmacopeial Convention, Inc.

American Institute of the History of Pharmacy
Madison, Wisconsin
1989

I.S.B.N. 0-931292-21-2

Publication No. 12 (New Series)
Gregory J. Higby and Elaine C. Stroud, General Editors

COVER: "Official Copy" stamp from the first combined NF/USP publication in 1980. The first such stamps appeared in the NF and the USP after the 1906 Act made them official. The 1985 revision of the NF/USP omits the stamp and includes the "official copy number" on the spine instead.

A Fischelis Publication
on Recent History and Trends of Pharmacy

third of a series aided by a fund established
in the American Institute of the History of Pharmacy

by

ROBERT P. FISCHELIS (1891–1981)

pharmacist · administrator · author · educator

Contents

Introduction

by Gregory J. Higby, Chairman

American pharmacy has changed dramatically during the last one hundred and fifty years, yet one overriding concern has remained unaltered: the accurate composition of medicines dispensed. Since 1906 the United States has been in the unique position of having two official compendia of drug standards, the *United States Pharmacopeia* and the *National Formulary*. Today they are merged in a single volume, with the differences between them realized only by specialists. Their origins, however, are vastly different and reveal something about the changing nature of drug standardization and American pharmacy. The USP was founded in 1820 by a convention of physicians interested in achieving some uniformity in the drugs and medicines being prepared by an emerging class of druggists and pharmacists. Although pharmacists participated in subsequent revisions of the USP, physicians were the dominant force in standardization for the next fifty years. In the 1880s two significant changes occurred: the task of revising the Pharmacopeia passed into the hands of pharmaceutical experts and the American Pharmaceutical Association published the first *National Formulary*.

To celebrate the first century of the *National Formulary*, a symposium was held on 13 March 1988 in Atlanta, Georgia. Co-sponsored by the American Institute of the History of Pharmacy and the United States Pharmacopeial Convention, Inc., the symposium appropriately took place at an annual meeting of the American Pharmaceutical Association, where, a century before, the membership had first heard of the early success of their first publication project. As the first paper in this volume shows, the first NF was not conceived as a compendium of drug standards or as another formula book, but as a weapon in the pharmacy profession's battle against ready made preparations and prescription medicines. The leadership of the American Pharmaceutical Association hoped that a recipe book of commonly made preparations would inspire physicians to write out complete prescriptions rather than order mass manufactured medicines.

After the NF was founded, however, it underwent rapid change. The second paper by Glenn Sonnedecker looks at the changing character of the National Formulary from 1890 to 1970. Not only did the outward appearance of the book and its monographs change, but so did the purpose and direction of the NF as well. As the modern NF became more and more like the USP in style and content, voices were raised that questioned the need for two separate compendia. Edward Feldmann shares his insights into the circumstances surrounding the NF-USP merger in the third paper in this booklet. As has been the case so often in the history of American pharmacy, threats from outside of the profession inspired pharmacy to action. Lastly, William Heller rounds out the symposium by detailing the NF-USP merger and speaking to the issue of the future of the National Formulary within America's voluntary system of standard setting.

As a supplement to the symposium, the preface and some selected monographs from the first *National Formulary* are included in this booklet. The basic character of NFI was straightforward and unpretentious. The first half of each monograph was aimed at physicians, with plenty of synonyms provided to encourage prescribing; the second half contained preparation instructions for the pharmacist. Often in the case of potent medicines the resultant strength of the active drug was included for the information of both professions. The important role played by the elixir craze in the birth of the NF is evident, with eighty-six recipes included in NFI for those preparations. As the full page of *errata* indicates, the APhA rushed to publish the long-awaited first edition of the *National Formulary.*

The idea for this symposium first arose in conversations between Roy Bowers, Executive Secretary of the Institute, and Joseph Valentino, Executive Associative of the USP. The success of the symposium is owed largely to the aid of its co-sponsor, USPC, Inc., Executive Director William Heller and Professional Affairs Director Alice Kimball. The Institute expresses appreciation to them for all their help and encouragement.

Publication of the National Formulary:
A Turning Point for American Pharmacy

by Gregory J. Higby

It is most appropriate that we come together in a room at an annual meeting of the American Pharmaceutical Association to commemorate the centennial of the National Formulary. At just such a meeting, in Detroit, on September 3, 1888, the Association learned of the surprising success of its first book publication. Copies of the book were not available to new members attending their first Association meeting, since the first three printings of 3000 each had been rapidly exhausted. The first run sold out in just ten days.[1] Quite an achievement when you consider the membership of the Association in 1888 was about 1300.

The publication of the *National Formulary* by the American Pharmaceutical Association in July of 1888 marks a turning point in the history of that organization and American pharmacy as a whole. It signaled the end of one era and the beginning of another. During the early nineteenth century, pharmacy arose in the USA as an independent profession out of the old wholesale drug trade. The foundation of the profession was the accurate compounding and dispensing of prescriptions from ingredients and standard preparations made and kept by the pharmacist. The ingredients and preparations recognized as necessary for a complete pharmacy practice were called "officinal." The objective of the United States Pharmacopoeia was to provide standards for these officinals. Opium, for example, was an officinal drug, with laudanum included as an officinal preparation. Preparations not included in the Pharmacopeia were referred to as "unofficinal" preparations, hence the peculiar title you find on the titlepage of the first *National Formulary.*

With those confusing terms out of the way, let us now turn to the founding of the National Formulary: what it reveals about American pharmacy and a few myths that have clung to the National Formulary over the years. No matter what the National Formulary became during the twentieth century, it was first established in the 1880s by pharmacists who had specific ideas of its concept and mission. The National Formulary was not just another in a long line of formula books published since the early days of the Republic. It was not connected directly with earlier efforts by the APhA to compile lists of formulas. And lastly, the National Formulary was not founded as a way station for old preparations or drugs on their destination of obscurity. Instead it was a book with a mission, a mission that it failed to accomplish. And like so many other failures, the National Formulary adapted and evolved into a success much greater than its creators could have imagined.

Chronology of the NF Founding

The main credit for founding the National Formulary belongs to one man, Charles Rice, the scholarly hospital pharmacist who also led the effort to modernize the Pharmacopeia of the United States. In September of 1885, he went to the Pittsburgh meeting of the APhA hoping that the Association would agree to adopt his plan for a new publication of unofficinal formulas. He came within a hair's breadth of failure. But that is getting a bit ahead of the story.

Space does not permit a full review of American publications containing a significant number of formulas, like William Buchan's *Domestic Medicine*,[2] or an examination of the impact of early military formularies, like the so-called Lititz Pharmacopoeia of 1778 and Coste's *Compendium Pharmaceuticum* of 1780, or hospital formularies like that of the New York Hospital published in 1811. Instead, I will turn directly to the sources of the National Formulary,

Gregory J. Higby, Ph.D., *is the Director of the American Institute of the History of Pharmacy and Adjunct Assistant Professor in the history of pharmacy at the University of Wisconsin-Madison. He received his doctorate at the University of Wisconsin (1984) in the history of pharmacy under the supervision of Glenn Sonnedecker. Although interested in all aspects of the history of pharmacy, Dr. Higby has concentrated his research efforts on the professional development of American pharmacy during the period 1820 to 1920.*

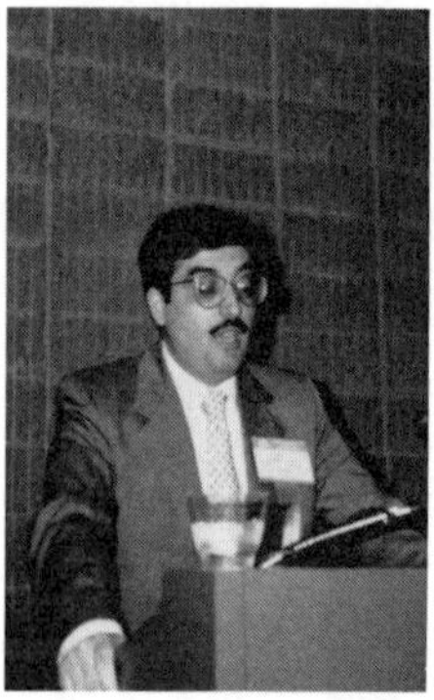

which have much to tell us about the nature of American pharmacy and its professional organizations during the Gilded Age.

Collection of Local Formulas

When the American Pharmaceutical Association was founded in Philadelphia in 1852, its charter members expressed no interest in collecting or publishing formulas for non-officinal preparations. They were concerned with the wide variation in quality that existed among imported drugs, as well as among practitioners of pharmacy.[3]

Pharmacy was struggling to gain some level of professional stature. During the 1820s and 1830s, physicians had increasingly turned over the compounding and dispensing of medicines to individuals trained in the art of pharmacy. A wide variety of factors contributed to this shift in professional roles: the growth in the number of drugs and preparations, the specialization of retail businesses, and the rapid increase in the number of school-trained physicians with scant experience in compounding. Pharmacists banded together to form

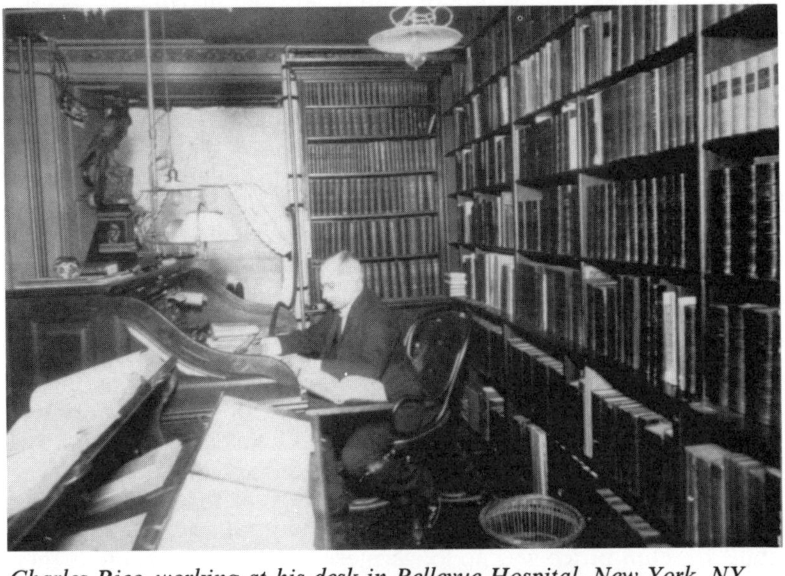

Charles Rice, working at his desk in Bellevue Hospital, New York, NY. Despite the hectic schedule at Bellevue Hospital, Rice found time to work on the revision of the United States Pharmacopoeia *and to keep up his study of Oriental languages (racks specially designed to hold his Sanskrit lexicon are in the front left of this photo). Rice was the first pharmacist to act as Chairman of the Revision Committee of the USP, and practically all the work related to this office was carried out here in his library at Bellevue. (Courtesy Kremers Reference Files, University of Wisconsin School of Pharmacy, Madison, WI.)*

local professional societies to share experiences and information about their art. Their occupational identity centered on their skills in manufacturing the basic or officinal ingredients needed in the making of medicines and the special knowledge necessary to compound the complex prescriptions of the day.

Uniformity, of course, was a prime concern of the young APhA. For this reason it reaffirmed again and again its support for the Pharmacopeia. The collection of unofficinal formulas, however, was not viewed as part of this effort. For that reason the young APhA took a rather relaxed approach to the subject. At the 1854 meeting of the Association two members submitted some local unofficinal formulas to the convention, which were to "be preserved by the Secretary, with a view to publication when future similar contributions accumulate sufficiently to justify it."[4]

One of those men was John Meakim of New York. He was a bit put off by this haphazard approach and at an Association meeting two years later in 1856, he put forward a successful motion that formed a committee charged with the "compilation of unofficinal formulae in local use with many physicians of our Union."[5] As the squeaky wheel, Meakim was named chairman of the committee. Over the next two years, the committee came up with a variety of formulas for liniments, pills, drops, plasters, and other mixtures.[6] Yet, these formulas were apparently not well received. As one committee report noted, "it is not the purpose of the Association to encourage the accumulation of unofficinal formulae, over the more explicit prescription of the physician."[7] And in 1858, the Committee on Local Unofficinal Formulae was discontinued.

The APhA's first effort to collect unofficinal formulas had a limited purpose and lifespan, and did not appeal much to the leadership of the Association. They had more pressing issues to contend with and *there was no strong need for a set of such formulas.* Formula books were a popular genre, with scores of titles appearing in English during the 1840s and 1850s.[8] Some of these, of course, were mere scissor and paste compilations. A few, like Robert E. Griffith's *A Universal Formulary*, were carefully prepared and documented. The objective of the APhA committee was to pull together *local* formulas, those that perhaps had slipped past other authors. Once done, the committee was no longer necessary. This early effort then was not the source of the National Formulary.

Rise of the Elixir

It was not until after the Civil War that changes within the American drug trade caused pharmacy organizations to again grapple with the issue of unofficinal formulas. Large-scale manufacturers who had thrived during war-time conditions, sought new markets at war's end, and discovered a ready demand for mass-manufactured drugs and preparations for use in compounding prescriptions. Leading pharmacists resisted this trend, arguing to physicians that preparations freshly produced in pharmacies made better prescriptions. Local pharmacy organizations in Baltimore and Newark published pamphlets with suggested recipes to be used by physicians. They hoped that physicians would write out the suggested recipes rather than call for ready-made preparations.[9]

The hopes of pharmacists that proprietaries were just a fad were dashed, however, when elixirs became the rage during the late 1860s and into the 1870s. Sweet, hydro-alcoholic preparations of bitter drugs, these fifty proof "medicines" gained a rapid popularity.[10] Prof. Faris Moore described the situation in 1872:

> The manufacturers canvass the country, visit every physician, make him a present of samples, and give him to understand that the preparation is to be had at every respectable drug store. The consequence is, the physicians prescribe them, and although the pharmacist may have a better article and all the talent to make what is necessary, he is compelled to keep a dozen kinds of the same elixir . . . to fill . . . prescriptions.[11]

The "elixir swindle" as it became known swept the nation during the early 1870s. Pharmacists were frustrated. Physicians claimed they had a simple choice—prescribe the old "nauseous solutions" their neighborhood druggists put up, or prescribe the new, pleasant-tasting elixirs made by large companies, and enjoyed by patients.[12] As one pharmacist put it, "the style of those medicines is so attractive that nearly the whole of the materia medica is drawn into the current of the elixir swindle."[13]

For American pharmacists of the early 1870s, the rapid rise in the prescribing of ready-made medicines threatened the professional progress they had worked so hard to achieve. At that time pharmacy in the United States was almost totally unregulated. Pharmacists did not have to have a diploma from a pharmacy school or a registration certificate on the wall of their shop. Anyone with sufficient capital and nerve could open a pharmacy. Only the work of their hands and their personal integrity demonstrated their professionalism.[14]

Quite simply, American pharmacy was facing the blossoming of modern pharmaceutical marketing. The remarks quoted from Prof. Moore are from a general discussion that followed a paper on the quality of some commercial elixirs. In that discussion, *for the first time,* the members of the Association grappled with the germs of problems that would burden the profession for the next century: drug efficacy, compliance, prescription drug advertising, sampling, trademarks, and substitution.[15]

To meet this challenge, the American Pharmaceutical Association appointed a committee "to take into consideration the subject of elixirs and similar unofficinal preparations, in all its bearings upon pharmacy, and if deemed proper, to report suitable formulas for the guidance of the members of this Association."[16] Concerned and conservative men, the leaders of the APhA were not seeking innovation, but instead a way to turn back the clock. If physicians were going to continue to prescribe elixirs, the APhA wanted them to write out the recipes rather than simply ask for something like *Compound Elixir of Cinchona, Stearns.*

The committee followed the approach advocated by C. Lewis Diehl of Louisville of using a basic Simple Elixir of one half ounce spirit of orange, four ounces of stronger alcohol, six ounces of cinnamon water, and six ounces of simple syrup. To this could be added an active ingredient, such as Cmpd Tinct of Cinchona, USP, to make Compd Elixir of Cinchona.

The elixir committee was uncomfortable with their task and asked to be relieved of it the next year, in 1873. The tone of their report is distainful of the entire subject, comparing elixirs with "nostrums," "the 'Mithridate' of old," and "placebos." Their work was frustrating in that their test preparations never matched the elegance of the large manufacturers, who, in the committee's words, "excelled us in the art of completely masking bitterness, . . . possibly [because] the active principles [are] only represented by the label."[17] The committee report was accepted, with copies sent to all American medical societies.[18]

From 1873–1875 the APhA and other pharmacy organizations struggled with the problem of the rapidly growing number of ready-made preparations, especially elixirs. Local organizations like the Chicago College of Pharmacy and the National College of Pharmacy in Washington, DC, proposed lists of formulas.[19] At annual meetings of the APhA in 1874 and 1875, discussions concerning elixir formulas became rather heated. Nomenclature posed a definite problem, since the various collections of formulas often carried local names, like "Dr. Smith's Cough Elixir," and reflected local preferences and tastes. Some Association members even objected to publishing the reports of their own committees, fearing that this would give official sanction to the "elixir swindle."[20]

Pharmacists were in a bind, with two great difficulties to solve: How to design elixir formulas that were both "elegant" and potent; and, most importantly, how to convince physicians to prescribe those formulas rather than ready-made elixirs. Over two hundred pharmacists who were not members of the APhA wrote to its secretary, John Maisch, asking for the Association's elixir formulas that had been published as a sixteen-page pamphlet in 1873. Many wrote back in disappointment at the poor quality of the elixirs produced according to those directions. One member commented that he had "heard considerable ridicule thrown upon the Association in consequence of those formulas" and urged that the Association avoid endorsing specific recipes.[21]. Apparently frustrated by the unceasing growth in the number and variety of elixirs and similar preparations, the APhA turned away from the subject for a few years.

At the 1880 annual meeting of the APhA, R. W. Gardner of New York began his contributed paper on "Elixirs and their Preparation" with the acknowledgment that: "some members of this Association are much averse to having this subject discussed at our meetings, and I am at a loss to account for it."

A laboratory manager for the Schieffelin firm, Gardner prepared formulas for thirty-five elixirs with obvious effort. Most of his elixirs contained four or more flavorings carefully balanced to counteract the negative flavor characteristics of each specific active ingredient. His elaborate formulations, arising from a commercial lab bench, elicited the opposite effect he sought. No discussion followed the presentation of his paper. Perhaps the high level of sophistication of his elixirs demonstrated to most members that such preparations were best manufactured where economies of scale permitted the cost-effective production of elegant pharmaceuticals, and that corner drug stores could not compete[22]

The Association published Mr. Gardner's recipes without adopting or recommending them. Perhaps they remembered what a member had said in 1875 about how people were ridiculing the Association for approving the formulas of the 1873 committee—that member had been R. W. Gardner!

The Spark for the National Formulary

No, the National Formulary did not spring from the efforts of the Meakim Committee of 1856 or the Hancock Committee of 1873 or any of the several committees on Unofficinal Formulae that existed between 1856 and 1880. The seed that grew into the National Formulary we are here to celebrate was planted on November 23, 1882, by an otherwise obscure New York pharmacist. On that date a special meeting of the New York College of Pharmacy was held to fill a recent vacancy on its board. As was usually the case in the winter months, a conversational meeting of the College also was held. Members gathered that night to discuss the new USP, which was causing quite a stir. There had been a dramatic shift in the nature and character of the Pharmacopeia from the previous revision.

No doubt the assembled group was glad to hear that Samuel Bendiner had brought along a short paper to read. Born in Budapest, Hungary, and educated in Vienna, Bendiner was well known among his colleagues for his wit and vigorous violin playing.[23] Bendiner did not disappoint them with his paper on "Manufacturers of Pharmaceutical Preparations: A Blessing and A Curse."[24] With sharp irony, he described the dependence of incompetent frontier doctors and druggists on proprietary elixirs. They could not write or compound a true prescription to save their lives. Bendiner's audience was doubtless amused.

With his colleagues off guard, Bendiner turned his attention to the cities of the East. Urban pharmacists had a legitimate gripe about the necessity of stocking several brands of the same preparation. But, in Bendiner's words "the most demoralizing fact resulting from this ever-increasing deluge of ready-made medicines . . . is that our assistants and eventual successors in business, and the students of pharmacy in this very building, whose standard of intellectual requirements is raised from year to year in correspondence with the rapid progress in all branches of our profession, and who, after examination, increase our ranks,—that all these aspiring disciples of knowledge are forced more and more into mental lithargy, as their task now mostly consists in taking a number of this man's coated pills or that firm's elixir, put in box or bottle, as the case may require, and write directions upon the label!

"That these lamentable conditions may not continue to that enormous extent, let us, educated pharmacists, appeal in a courteous spirit to the educated physicans to stop prescribing ready-made medicines of doubtful value, and thereby maintain our interests and the dignity of our profession as they maintain their own."[25]

During the discussion that followed, Bendiner suggested that a committee be formed to compile a formulary of unofficinal preparations for the New York area.[26] Inspired by Mr. Bendiner's rhetoric, a committee of three was appointed to draft a circular "calling the attention of the medical fraternity to the subject."[27]

Like a prophet of old, Bendiner chastised his brethren into action that led eventually to the founding of the National Formulary, even though the disaster he predicted—the advent of count and pour pharmacy—could not be avoided.

The ad hoc committee was organized permanently on April 27, 1883, as the Committee on Formulae for Elixirs and Similar Preparations, with the eminent P. W. Bedford as chairman of the five-man group.[28] As an active member of the New York German Apothecaries' Society, Bendiner got them involved as well. With members of the nearby Kings County Pharmaceutical Society added, a combined committee began work on compiling a manual of formulas.

There was nothing exceptional in this local effort to put together a formulary of unofficinal preparations. One of the first activities of the young Philadelphia College of Pharmacy in 1828, was the publication of a pamphlet listing recipes of popular patent medicines. Other local or state pharmaceutical associations published formula books throughout the middle half of the nineteenth century. What made the New York and Brooklyn formulary effort special was that among the representatives from the New York German Apothecaries' Society was a gentleman named Charles Rice, who had been, among other things, the chairman of the Revision Committee of the 1880 USP.

Perhaps inspired by the example of the New York group, the APhA appointed a new committee on unofficinal formulas at its 1883 meeting. This committee, however, was composed of gentlemen scattered about the nation, and thus had a great deal of difficulty working together. When the time came to report at the 1884 APhA meeting, they were unable to deliver a set of formulas. Their chairman did allude to the *New York and Brooklyn Formulary,* which had appeared a few months earlier.[29] Peter Bedford, chairman of the New York committee, passed along to the APhA that all were free to use the *New York and Brooklyn Formulary,* but not to reprint it. They had gone to considerable expense to finish and publish the project and so had copyrighted it. This action, however, had made it, in the view of the APhA leadership, impossible for the Association to adopt the NY and Brooklyn formulas as official.[30]

To break the impass that they seemed to face, the APhA came up with a novel solution: it appointed a totally new committee on unofficinal formulas, composed of five members from the joint committee that had put together the *New York and Brooklyn Formulary.* Desperate to get action on a problem that had beset the Association on and off for decades, the APhA cast aside any pretence of a truly "national" committee, chosing instead the sort of local working group that had been used so successfully in the past for revising the Pharmacopeia.[31]

This focussed activity occurred in late August of 1884, but the first *National Formulary* did not come off the presses until July of 1888, nearly four years later. A look at this delay reveals much about the still immature American Pharmaceutical Association.

Delays in Organizing

During 1884 and early 1885 the *New York and Brooklyn Formulary* attracted much attention and good reviews. The *Druggists' Circular* carried extracts from it in several issues, as well as reports that New York area pharmacists had used the new formulary to obtain authorized substitutions of in-shop preparations for commercial elixirs.[32]

Meanwhile, the combined committee of the NYCP, Kings County Pharmaceutical Society and the New York German Apothecaries' Society, continued to meet and work on revising their formulary. It was Charles Rice's hope that the efforts of this large committee could serve as the working basis for a national formulary.

When Charles Rice came to the APhA meeting in Pittsburgh in September of 1885, he carried an unusual three-point proposition from the three New York-area pharmaceutical societies:

1. The joint committee of the New York and Brooklyn formulary would hand over their formulary to the APhA to be used as the basis of a national formulary.

2. The three NY Societies would continue to hold copyright over the formulary until the Association was ready to take it over, or the three societies would hold copyright jointly with the APhA if so desired by the Association.

3. The joint committee would turn over papers and records concerning their work to the Association. The committee also suggested that they be retained as the editing committee of the national formulary.

After giving his formal report as chairman of the APhA committee on unofficinal formulas, Rice explained that the copyright issue came up because the Association was not incorporated and therefore unable to hold copyright. He hoped that some arrangement could be made between the New York societies and the Association.

While APhA members all spoke highly of the New York Formulary, some, led by Albert Ebert, opposed the APhA getting into the publishing business or holding a copyright. The Association could only hold a copyright if it incorporated and Ebert opposed that as well. Caught up in this issue, the body of the Association seemed to be moving away from Rice's proposal. Rice stepped in, trying to save what seemed to be a dying proposal. Usually softspoken, Rice saw his dream slipping away, and, according to witnesses, grew visibly anxious and disconcerted.

You see Rice came to Pittsburgh with more than just a set of proposals. As head of the Revision Committee of the USP, Rice hoped that the Association's formulary would serve as a repository for the poly-pharmaceuticals he wanted expunged from the Pharmacopeia. He did not want complex elixirs, no matter how potent or popular, in his USP. Using the *New York and Brooklyn Formulary* as a foundation, Rice aimed to design a national formulary that would be a sort of semi-official, secondary pharmacopoeia.[33]

The haggling over the good and bad of publishing a national formulary separate from the Association proceedings took a long time by Association standards. Joseph Remington got the floor, pointed out the time lost and the entire subject was deferred. Rice's national formulary seemed jeopardized.[34]

That may have been the case a few years before, but in 1885 the Association membership was convinced that the elixir and proprietary situation was getting out of control. Something had to be done.[35]

So after that day's session, some late night negotiating went on. Ebert, who had led the earlier opposition, got the floor early the next morning and made a motion to *accept* the offer from the NY societes, publish the *New York and Brooklyn Formulary* in the APhA proceedings, with the intention that it serve as the basis for a national formulary. And further, Ebert moved that when complete, the National Formulary "be published by the American Pharmaceutical Association in such a form as to place it within easy reach of all pharmacists.[36]

Rice was relieved. He took the floor and rambled through a nervous recap of what had occurred. Fortunately his plan was not going to be rejected and his hopes for a secondary pharmacopeia were still alive. Ebert's motion carried unanimously, as did another that the 1884 committee on the Report of Unofficinal Formulas, chaired by Rice, be reappointed.

The National Formulary committee set to work right after the APhA meeting concluded in Pittsburgh. They usually met two or three times a month, spending most of their time evaluating the formulas sent in by individuals, and state and local pharmaceutical associations. Again, the work was done largely by the five-man committee, with aid from other pharmacists from the three New York area societies.[37]

When the 1886 APhA meeting opened in Providence, Rhode Island, on September 7, President Joseph Roberts of Baltimore began his presidential address attacking the "large and increasing demand for proprietary medicines, which filches from the pharmacist so large a portion of his legitimate profits."[38] These laments were reiterated by the Report on the Drug Market.[39]

Charles Rice's report as Chairman of the NF committee reveals that he had expanded his working group to twenty—the five appointed by the Association, plus five each from the New York College of Pharmacy, the Kings County Pharmaceutical Society, and the New York German Apothecaries Society. The matter of scope was decided by the committee to include "every preparation legitimately belonging to pharmacy which is in professional or popular demand" not in the USP or purely trivial.[40]

Acknowledging the decision of the USP to use a system of parts by weight rather than conventional weights and measures in its next revision, the National Formulary committee decided not to follow the USP and adopt definite weights and measures. This decision probably reflects Rice's own view of this metrology controversy.[41] To avoid problems with nomenclature, Latin titles were given to all the formulas, with synonyms below.

As had been the case at the 1885 meeting, Rice came to the 1886 meeting with an elaborate set of propositions for approval by the assembled membership. They included that the National Formulary could contain formulas that had been or could be officinal in the USP or other pharmacopeias; that the National Formulary use standard apothecaries' weights and measures, only using parts by weight when convenient, as with ointments; that the National Formulary committee have complete charge of publishing the book, from start to finish, before turning over its duties to a new committee.[42]

After much talk and almost no change, Rice's propositions were adopted with the rest of the National Formulary committee report, but he got more than he bargained for.[43]

The next day a motion was passed to place one person from each state pharmaceutical association on the National Formulary committee, in addition to the five already appointed, with five serving as a quorum. The objective: to make the National Formulary as "national as possible." Rice acquiesced. The idea was fine with him as long as it was understood that the five New York members could decide all issues alone.

As in the previous year, the Proceedings for 1886 contained a collection of formulas—this being a *Preliminary Draft of a National Formulary of Unofficinal Preparations.* Significantly different from the old *New York and Brooklyn Formulary,* this draft had the arrangement, format, and "feel" of what came to be known as the NF.

When the APhA gathered for its thirty-fifth annual meeting in 1887, the situation with manufactured drugs had not improved. The normally staid reporter on the progress of pharmacy, C. Lewis Diehl of Louisville, began his report with a rather poetic look at the growth of medicinal specialties, as he called trade products. In his words, "most of these specialties [are] based upon false premises, false representations, and false conclusions. . . . What the future of pharmacy will be has puzzled the wisest of the profession. Just as the development of manufacturing facilities has taken the preparation of chemicals from the hands of the pharmacists, so will eventually the manufacture of galenical preparations that require more than ordinary attention be taken away."[44]

Once again when the report of the Committee on the National Formulary was read it asked for more time and contained five propositions for the attention of the assembled membership. The important points in these propositions were that the present committee be retained, that the NF not be issued as part of the Proceedings, and that a new formulary committee be appointed at the next APhA meeting. This new committee should be from a different part of the country to gain a new viewpoint.[45] Their hope was that the NF would be finished by 1 March 1888 and a copy sent to every member who received the proceedings.[46]

The discussion that followed included some strong criticism from C. S. N. Hallberg that the NF was not going to include the leading proprietary preparations of the West, while including "at least 50 or 60 old elixirs, and about 40 of the syrups" that were hardly used any more. Members rushed to Rice's defense, including Remington who said that "Doctor Charles Rice has done everything an honest man could do." And the committee report and propositions were approved.[47]

At later meetings of the APhA Council, the issue of copyright was discussed. By a vote of seven to one a motion to copyright passed, with Albert Ebert still opposed to the idea. Because of this motion a special committee of three was appointed to consider the question of incorporation, necessary for copyrighting.[48]

During a paper session at this 1887 meeting, long-time member Emlen Painter read a paper on "The Medicines of Medicine" where he estimated the extent of the pharmaceutical manufacturing in the USA. "There are in the United States not less than 160 different so-called 'manufacturers of pharmaceutical preparations,' who in reality, for the most part, are but mere manipulators and mixers of drugs. At least 25 per cent of this number have offices in New York, and a still larger percentage send out their drummers to the medical men in this vicinity to distribute samples, to extol their wares, and to urge the physician to designate their particular 'make' in prescribing." According to Painter those forty-odd manufacturers listed a total of 36,500 mixtures![49]

The NF is Published

As had been the case, the NF committee was a bit optimistic about the timetable it could follow. Rather than meeting the March 1, 1888, deadline set for it by the Association, the Editing Committee finally pushed the Formulary through the presses on July 2, 1888. The dues paying membership of about 1300 received the first copies, with additional orders following.

When the Association met in September of 1888 in Detroit, they immediately turned to the issue of revising the National Formulary. The Rice Committee participated in this discussion, but was glad to be relieved of its duties,[50] nearly six years after their formulary work began. Rice estimated that from 1885 to 1888 he had spent one and a half hours every day on NF work.

Conclusion

Sparked by the witty remarks of a Hungarian-American pharmacist, a stuttering, drawn-out process eventually led to the founding of a new American institution, the National Formulary. Historians have had the tendency to lump it together with the plethora of recipe books of the time or to see it as merely the USP's backdoor to therapeutic oblivion. In the pages that follow others will comment on what the NF became, so I will limit myself to the significance of its founding.

First, the development and publication of the NF forced the APhA to mature. Up until 1888, the Association had been an *ad hoc* organization, which existed for the purpose of holding an annual meeting and sharing pertinent information through its published proceedings. With only two significant continuing officers—a corresponding secretary and a reporter on the Progress of Pharmacy—the APhA of the 1870s and 1880s was an organization in relative decline, in both membership and influence. State pharmaceutical associations, which were largely founded during this period to facilitate the passage of state practice acts and the establishment of pharmacy schools, attracted far more members. In 1885, for example, the state pharmaceutical associations of New York and Pennsylvania combined had more members than the entire APhA. Only about one in twenty pharmacists belonged to the APhA, while membership in state and local organizations was closer to one in five. With the NF came the need to incorporate, establish more permanency, and forge links with pharmacists throughout the nation who would buy and distribute the Association's first book publication.

Second, the NF should not be viewed as the inevitable product of several abortive efforts to put together a collection of unofficinal formulas. The efforts by the APhA in the 1850s and 1870s to collect formulas did not eventually lead to the NF. These were attempts to gather local formulas for the purpose of sharing information—a central purpose of the Association. The committees issued reports on local unofficinal preparations. The NF was conceived separately and distinctly from these previous efforts. With the chairman of the Revision Committee of the Pharmacopoeia at its head, the NF committee had the wherewithal and authority to claim its national status.

Third, no matter what the NF became, it was not conceived or established as a repository for old USP drugs. Rice did hide his intention to move polypharmaceutical preparations out of the USP and into the NF, but the evidence shows that the NF was far from a dumping ground. Of the 435 formulas included, only four were discards from USP 1870 or USP 1880.

No, instead the NF was devised to treat an ailment that was weakening American pharmacy and threatening its professional life—the rise of the manufacturing of ready-made medicines and proprietary drugs for prescriptions. American pharmacy was going through a transitional phase from an older model of professionalism based on individual demonstration of skill and honesty to the modern form of professionalism based on paper credentials such as diplomas and registration certificates. For the professionally-minded APhA member of 1888, in-house manufacture of preparations was the prime foundation of their professionalism. Dispensing ready-made medicines made them mere shop keepers. They, of course, were a small minority of practitioners; many, if not most of the vast majority of less educated pharmacists probably welcomed the appearance of trade products as time-saving, at least in the late 1860s and early 1870s.

The efforts of the APhA to do something about the elixir swindle during the 1870s probably failed because the threat was just to the professional status of pharmacists. By the 1880s, however, the number of different elixirs had decreased, but the number of manufacturers had burgeoned. The issue shifted from professional outrage—"I can make anything XYZ & Co. can make and better!" to one of sheer commercialism—"I'm sick of carrying five different brands of Compound Elixir of Cinchona!" The APhA responded to this widespread call for help with the NF, and American pharmacy reacted positively. Membership, which had dropped during the mid-1880s, increased after 1888.

Lastly, of course, is the issue of effectiveness. Did the NF cure the blight of proprietaries? No, it did not. This becomes evident if we compare two prescription surveys done before and after the publication of the first NF. According to the 1885 Ebert survey of about 16,000 prescriptions, approximately 54% of the ingredients were official in USP VI, with 39% being unofficinal and 7% being proprietary items. The 1895 survey done by C. S. N. Hallberg found 51% of the ingredients being official, with 27% unofficinal, 14% proprietary, and 7% from NF I.[51]

The basic problem with the effectiveness of the NF was that it relied on the interest and effort of physicians primarily. Unless a pharmacist could convince his local physicians to either call for NF preparations or allow the pharmacist the right to substitute, the goal was lost. Unfortunately for pharmacy, the manufacturers had hundreds of drummers and thousands of dollars of advertising at their disposal. A thin little book did not stand much of a chance. Nevertheless it marked a changing focus for pharmacy.

The title of this paper promises a turning point. For American pharmacy the publication of the National Formulary marks the point where the great compounding debate formally begins. With the 1880 revision of the USP supervised by Rice, the standards for officinal drugs were changed to reflect the reality that the basic ingredients for prescriptions were mainly mass-produced rather than made in shop. All but a few of the old guard accepted this development graciously. The compounding of prescriptions, however, was a different matter. That was the heart and soul of pharmacy. The appearance of the elixirs and other trade products in the years following the Civil War heralded the onset of modern pharmacy and the beginning of the end of the compounding function of the pharmacist. At first, the profession ignored the problem, hoping it would be just a fad, a fancy. It was not. The profession's first action? The National Formulary, a book carefully conceived to hold off the torrent of elixirs.

As we know, it failed to hold back the flood. Yet it was not a total failure. Physicians did adopt many of the formulas and prescribe preparations with titles followed with "NF." More importantly, the National Formulary became much more than just a book of formulas to give to your neighborhood physicians to encourage "true" prescribing. It became an official compendium controlled by the pharmaceutical profession. But that is for the next paper to address.

Notes and References

1. *Proceedings of the American Pharmaceutical Association* 36 (1888): 29. Henceforth, the Proceedings will be abbreviated, *Proc. APhA*.
2. David L. Cowen, *America's Pre-Pharmacopoeial Literature* (AIHP, 1976), p. 16.
3. *Proc. APhA* (1852): 8–11.
4. *Proc. APhA* 3 (1854): 8.
5. *Proc. APhA* 5 (1856): 27.
6. "Report of the Committee on Local Unofficinal Formulae, &c.," *Proc. APhA* 6 (1857): 79–99.
7. Ibid., 79.
8. The catalog of the National Library Medicine reveals the titles of over one hundred formula or recipe books published in English from 1800 to 1850.
9. "Pharmaceutical Colleges and Associations," *American Journal of Pharmacy* 43 (1871): 278.
10. [William Procter, Jr.], "Editorial: Modern Elixirs," *American Journal of Pharmacy* 43 (1871): 332f.
11. *Proc. APhA* 20 (1872): 80.
12. Robert J. Brown, "Unofficinal Preparations," *Proc. APhA* 20 (1872): 207.
13. Ottmar Eberbach, "On the amount of alkaloids contained in some commercial elixirs," *Proc. APhA* 20 (1872): 264.
14. Gregory J. Higby, "Professionalism and the Nineteenth-Century American Pharmacist," *Pharmacy in History* 28 (1986): 115–124.
15. *Proc. APhA* 20 (1872): 80–85.
16. *Proc. APhA* 20 (1872): 111.
17. *Proc. APhA* 21 (1873): 116–117.
18. *Proc. APhA* 22 (1874): 573.
19. "[Review of] Formulae for non-officinal preparations in general use in the District of Columbia, 1875," *American Journal of Pharmacy* 48 (1876): 238–239.
20. *Proc. APhA* 22 (1874): 559–564; *Proc. APhA* 23 (1875): 775–776, 784–790.
21. *Proc. APhA* 23 (1875): 784f.
22. R. W. Gardner, "Elixirs and their Preparation," *Proc. APhA* 28 (1880): 439–453.
23. *Proc. APhA* 45 (1897): 33.
24. *Pharmaceutical Record* 3 (1883): 8.
25. Ibid., 8.
26. *Proc. APhA* 33 (1885): 558.
27. *Druggists Circular* 27 (1883): 12.
28. *Pharmaceutical Record* 3 (1883): 155.
29. *Druggists Circular* 28 (1884): 88.

30. *Proc. APhA* 32 (1884): 506–7.
31. Ibid., 508.
32. *Druggists Circular* 28 (1884): 88, 117; *Druggists Circular* 29 (1885): 21; *Am. J. Pharm.* 56 (1884): 348.
33. John Uri Lloyd, "What Should be the Scope of the next National Formulary?" *Bulletin of Pharmacy* 34 (1920): 96–97.
34. *Proc. APhA* 33 (1885): 564.
35. *Proc. APhA* 33 (1885): 541f.
36. *Proc. APhA* 33 (1885): 574.
37. *Pharmaceutical Record* 6 (1886): 2.
38. *Proc. APhA* 34 (1886): 129.
39. *Proc. APhA* 34 (1886): 1–2.
40. *Proc. APhA* 34 (1886): 159.
41. Ibid., 160. See also, Gregory J. Higby and Glenn Sonnedecker, "Adoption of the Metric System in the U. S. Pharmacopoeia," *Journal of the History of Medicine and Allied Sciences* 40 (1985): 207–213.
42. Ibid., 162–164.
43. *Proc. APhA* 34 (1886): 159–169.
44. *Proc. APhA* 35 (1887): 1–3.
45. *Proc. APhA* 35 (1887): 496–497.
46. *Proc. APhA* 35 (1887): 646.
47. *Proc. APhA* 35 (1887): 496–502.
48. *Proc. APhA* 35 (1887): 504.
49. *Proc. APhA* 35 (1887): 593–598.
50. *Proc. APhA* 36 (1888): 45–46.
51. E. N. Gathercoal, *The Prescription Ingredient Survey* (Washington, DC: APhA, 1933).

The Changing Character of the National Formulary (1890–1970)

by Glenn Sonnedecker

During the eighty-seven years that the National Formulary (NF) remained under the sponsorship of the American Pharmaceutical Association it underwent striking changes of character. A single event profoundly influenced the NF's evolution: Congressional enactment of the first Federal Food and Drugs Act, in June 1906. The law made even the title of the *National Formulary of Unofficinal Preparations* an anomaly when it designated the NF as an official source of enforceable specifications for drugs.[1]

The Pharmacopeia of the United States of America (USP) itself had no officiality as a legally enforceable standard before the Federal law of 1906, except in a few state statutes, although physicians and pharmacists for decades had termed the USP their "official" guide. This courtesy status was rooted in respect and in the presumed authority of democratically organized representatives of medicine and pharmacy in setting drug specifications. At least one state, Pennsylvania, had set a precedent by naming the NF as a legal standard alongside the USP as early as 1897.[2]

The founders of the unpretentious NF, however, had no ambitions toward "officiality." Those responsible for the NF said they "had not foreseen its adoption as a legal standard." A member of the NF Committee termed it "a most startling and unexpected occurrence" and said, "The change was such a sudden one and one so great in its consequences that comparatively few, even yet, realize what it means and how increased importance carries with it increased responsibilities and more exacting requirements."[3] How, then, did this curious surprise come about?

It is unclear; but James H. Beal, a pharmacist-lawyer involved in legislative affairs, said, "I have always given Dr. [Harvey] Wiley credit for their [i.e., the NF and USP's] original introduction into the various drafts." In considering the proposed food and drug legislation, the National Pure Food and Drug Congress (1898–1900) favored designating the NF an official standard; but Lyman F. Kebler recalled that the NF was added and deleted repeatedly from bills that preceded the 1906 enactment. According to Beal, "It was generally believed by the delegates to the Congress that the opposition to the N.F. was inspired wholly by the [pharmaceutical] manufacturers." Whatever the exact circumstance, the United States apparently became the only country in the world having *two* books legally recognized as standards for allopathic drugs.[4]

Pharmacists comprising the APhA seem to have had mixed feelings about the new status of one of their most ambitious projects. For example, the Committee on the President's Address in 1909 retorted to President Oscar Oldberg: "We find that part of the president's address referring to the National Formulary in which he states that Congress made a ridiculous mistake in adopting it as a legal standard is unwarranted, unjust and uncalled for." Some were concerned that the NF would become less practical, less a manual primarily for the practicing pharmacist.[5]

When NF III appeared in 1906, however, it was still cast in the original mold as a traditional formulary, fostering uniformity of composition and nomenclature for the compound medicines that it recognized, but devoid of the purity rubrics, tests, and other specifications that the USP had begun to introduce. Two years later the APhA adopted a series of revised principles that would guide

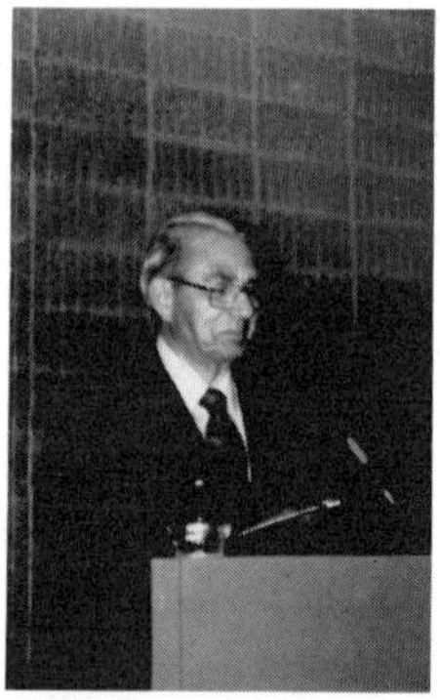

Glenn Sonnedecker, *Ph.D., received his doctorate under the guidance of the late pharmacist-historian George Urdang at the University of Wisconsin-Madison. Sonnedecker succeeded Urdang on the University's faculty as a historian of pharmacy and later became the second Director of the American Institute of the History of Pharmacy. Dr. Sonnedecker is currently Honorary Director of the AIHP, President of the International Academy of the History of Pharmacy, and Professor Emeritus of the University of Wisconsin. Among other honors and awards he has been the recipient of the Remington Honor Medal, the George Urdang Medal and Edward Kremers Award of the AIHP, and the Schelenz Plaquette of the International Society of the History of Pharmacy.*

changes in the character of the NF during the ensuing revision. The general thrust was to harmonize the NF with the activities and the character of the USP, while preserving the traditional conceptual difference between the two books—the USP setting specifications for drugs of first choice therapeutically, the NF for other drugs whose extent of use justified development of a monograph.

During the next several revisions the character of the NF became increasingly hard to distinguish from that of the USP, except for drug admission policy. Collaboration between the two works became increasingly close, if occasionally uncomfortable; governmental and industrial input became more frequent; the limited scientific facilities of the practicing pharmacist became less determinant in writing official specifications for each drug; pharmaceutical scientists rather than practitioners came to dominate the revision process; the customary ten-year revision cycle was cut to five years (formalized 1938), paralleling a new USP policy; and after Congressional enactment of the new Food, Drug and Cosmetic Act of 1938 and the Drug Amendments of 1962, the preoccupation with the legal implications of what was said between the covers of the NF (and of the USP) became even more pervasive.[6] Thus, during a quarter century, the *National Formulary* was transformed. Nowhere was this more striking than in the quantification of drug specifications.

Quantification of Standards

The original concept of the NF, reflected in the first three editions, placed in the hands of pharmacists formulas that could be compounded on a small scale, both to meet the wants of physicians and the wants of a self-medicating public. This type of formulary for hand-crafted medicines came out of a literary tradition stretching back to the earliest known pharmaceutical records.

The kinds of precise specifications for each substance that help assure purity, authenticity, and predictable therapeutic effect were simply not part of the mission of the early NF Committees. But even the first three editions had a standardizing influence in modest ways. For example, some formulas going into the NF had drifted through the medical community in several versions that varied the kinds or amounts of ingredients; and the identifying name of the product sometimes varied by region of the country. Against this tendency the NF Committee fostered uniformity of product by carefully specifying the kinds and amounts of ingredients, specifying a standard process of preparation, and specifying an appropriate name for each product in both Latin and English.

Yet, for the USDA Bureau of Chemistry charged with safeguarding the nation's drug supply under the 1906 Act, this approach soon came to seem insufficient. After all, Karl R. Fresenius had published his systematization of quantitative chemistry already in 1846; and in the United States Albert Lyons had published in 1886 his first *Manual of Practical Pharmaceutical Assaying* encouraging American drug makers to assay and adjust their products for strength and purity. One pharmacist-chemist of the government's Bureau of Chemistry, speaking of the NF in 1910, said that formula standardization alone was inadequate. "It would be far better," he told an APhA branch meeting, "to have a definite standard prescribed when practicable for each product recognized." Without standardization of both ingredients and conditions when preparing "Beef, Iron and Wine" (NF III, 1906), for example, the precipitate is a "variable quantity depending upon the temperature at the time of preparation, the alcoholic strength of the wine, and the character and quality of the beef extract used, with the result that the finished product is likewise of variable composition."[7]

The NF IV (1916) took a giant step in responding to such calls for setting "a definite standard." This can be seen clearly in a new Part II where the NF provided monographs for the "simples," that is, for the individual ingredients that entered into the compound medicaments of Part I (if the USP had not already provided specifications). In listing a botanical drug, for example, the NF IV provided concrete specification of the species and the part of the plant to be utilized, the permissible percentage of foreign matter, the odor, taste, and color, a description of the macroscopic and microscopic appearance, and so on. In listing a medicinal chemical the NF provided a physical description and empirical formula, a purity rubric, the melting point or boiling point, specific gravity, quantitative residues, and sometimes an assay.

If the NF sometimes seemed slow to adopt the most refined standards and advanced laboratory techniques for drug makers to use in checking their products, two factors played a part: First, the NF (and USP) standards had to hold up in a court of law as proved and reliable criteria for allegedly sub-standard medicaments; and, second, the requirements should not make an unreasonable demand on the small-scale drug manufacturer. The original intent that the NF would be a valued aid to the ordinary practitioners of pharmacy and of medicine was an intent not readily abandoned.

A harbinger that the future lay in a different direction appeared in 1925 when the new NF Chairman, Professor E. N. Gathercoal of Illinois, established a working relationship with large-scale pharmaceutical industry through a "Combined Pharmaceutical Contact Committee," which recently had been formed mainly to provide liaison between industry and the USDA Bureau of Chemistry. One of the first fruits of opening this channel of interaction between industrial laboratories and the NF Committee was a major improvement of the specifications in NF VI (1936) for injectable drugs and for tablets and capsules. Thus began the advisory contributions from the Contact Committee that appear to have been constructive on the technical side of the standard-setting process.

To generate new or improved testing procedures, drug formulas, or purity standards for each monograph, however, the NF would continue to rely upon a network of volunteers around the country in laboratories of universities and elsewhere. Some projects received small subsidies from the APhA (e.g., $4000 in 1936).[8] A structure of subcommittees and panels evolved within the NF Committee to evaluate data thus generated and to recommend what changes in the next edition the findings might imply.

This system was enhanced beginning in 1935 when an NF laboratory was set up at the University of Illinois College of Pharmacy, where Chairman Gathercoal was on the faculty. Three years later the APhA reestablished the laboratory, with a small full-time staff, in its new headquarters building in Washington.[9]

The structure of the NF monographs gradually became virtually indistinguishable from those of the USP. During the 1950s more sophisticated analytical techniques were made serviceable for determining the strength, quality, purity, and identity of drugs. These entered into a significant number of NF tests and assays for the first time in the Eleventh Edition (1960)—for example, nonaqueous ti-

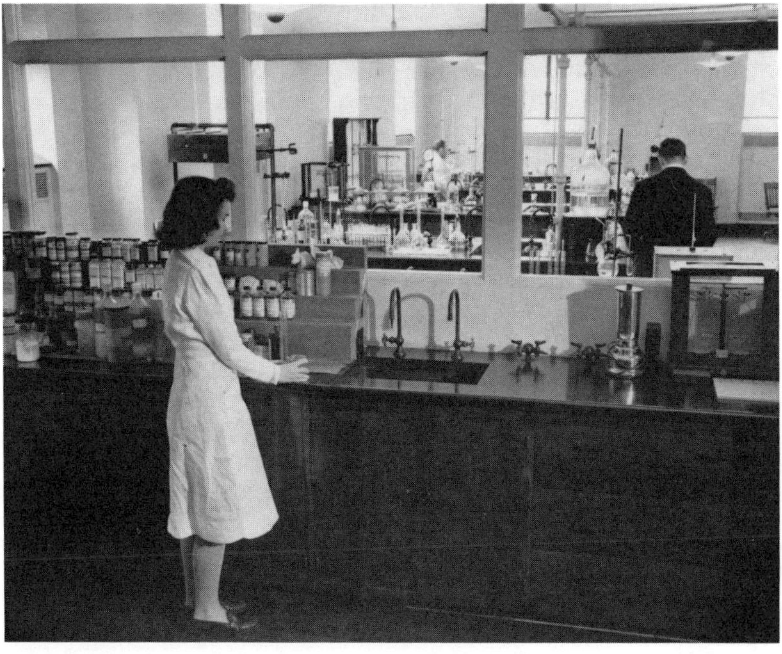

APhA Laboratory in 1944 during checks on standardization procedures for drugs to be included in NF VIII. (APhA photo)

trimetry, complexometry, ultraviolet and infrared spectrophotometry, and column and paper chromatography. To compensate for variation among instruments used for spectrophotometric assays, the NF had to increase four-fold the number of reference standards (i.e., drug samples certified as official) against which the mass-produced drugs could be compared.

Other new types of specifications were inaugurated in NF XII (1965). For example, a new requirement was adopted for demonstrating the content uniformity within a lot of tablets of any highly potent drug. The permissible disintegration times for various kinds of tablets were cut drastically, in most cases by at least 50%. For most timed-release medications, an assurance of product uniformity also was specified. Some of the assaying techniques specified for the first time reflect dramatic changes then taking place in quantification of standards, notably the use of gas-liquid chromatography, thin-layer chromatography, flame spectrophotometry, polarography, and delta-pH titrimetry. Assays were installed in a number of drug monographs that lacked such a criterion in earlier editions. Many of the identity tests and purity tests were improved.[10]

The industrial use of automated analytical procedures for some quality controls invoked new legal considerations in the 1960s. It was the kind of technologic advance that, if officially *required* by the NF (or USP), would be financially out of the question for small manufacturers. The NF response was to *permit* automation as an alternate procedure, if "employing the same basic chemistry as those procedures given in the monographs," and if it were understood that "only the result obtained by the procedure given in this National Formulary is authoritative" in case of doubt or dispute about a drug's conformity with standards.[11]

While preparing NF XIII (1970) a USP-NF Joint Panel on Physiological Availability was appointed to cope with a question increasingly raised: Which drugs, though they meet official standards, may vary enough in *physiologic* availability so that an additional dimension of quality specification need be devised? Two approaches introduced into NF XIII (1970) were a much more stringent dissolution test for tablets and capsules, and a requirement of conformity to a specified test pattern of X-ray diffraction when the tested substance occurs in variable crystal forms. The character of some NF monographs thus would take on a significant new dimension if accumulating research data proved that the physical characteristics of one of the officially recognized drugs presented a bioavailability problem.

By the end of the 1960s, the NF and USP alike had in place sophisticated checks on the quality of drugs that drastically improved their precision, accuracy, and selectivity, and permitted the testing of samples infinitely smaller than could be used previously.

Drugs and Dosage Forms of the NF

A predictable purity and strength of medicines remained high on a pharmacist's scale of values, though the scientific complexity of NF standards had removed even the possibility of applying them to products on the shelves of a local pharmacy.

Of equally durable interest was a question about *which* drugs should be recognized by the NF and dealt with in the monographs. The Pharmacopeia had stuck by its original concept of scope, recognizing only drugs of first choice in each therapeutic category, as determined by representatives of organized medicine. This left a majority of the medicaments open for selection by the NF, and left ample room for differences of opinion. The pharmacist's journals reflected this interest at least until industrialization removed drug manufacture and most compounding from the local pharmacy.

NF II (1896), like its predecessor, consisted entirely of multiple-ingredient formulas that an average pharmacist could utilize in a back-room laboratory. But large-scale laboratories already were flooding the market nationally with such products. Some practitioners felt that the NF was just what they needed to keep physicians prescribing—in the tried and true manner—products of known composition made by the pharmacist's own hand.

The idea that the NF would include many products not admissible by the selective USP was only partly outgrown during the decades that the NF remained under APhA sponsorship. One influential member of the NF Committee, Henry P. Hynson of Baltimore, said he did not "intend that the NF shall be the dumping ground for the rubbish of the Pharmacopoeia."[12] Wilbur L. Scoville contended "that it contains too many things which are of no value."[13]

The character of the NF eventually changed for the better by eliminating some products against which Hynson took specific aim. These included what he called, in 1910, "undignified" combinations (e.g., Camphor Ice, Tar Plaster, Aromatic Vinegar); old family remedies "not in accord with present therapeutic practice" (e.g., Godfrey's Cordial, Bateman's Drops, Warburg's Tincture); some formulas of "bad odor" (e.g., Compound Elixir of Celery, Chloroform Anodyne, Elixir of Cramp Bark); and objectionable polypharmacal preparations (e.g., Compound Syrup Actea, Compound Syrup of Wild Ginger, Decoction of Aloes).[14]

But the NF Committee's response was conservative and the issue chronic, for on principle the NF was committed to admissions based on extent of use, rather than therapeutic respectability. This policy was underpinned by a lingering precept that it was the pharmacist's responsibility to fulfill the complete medicinal needs of the community at a high level of quality, not to pass judgment on the therapeutic rationale. Still in NF V (1926) the original character of the book was retained, explicitly on grounds that it is "essentially a book of pharmaceutical formulas, selected on the basis of their use by physicians, but with no endorsement of their therapeutic worth."

With the appearance of NF VI (1936), it became evident that polypharmacal compounding no longer would dominate the character of the NF. Operative formulas were expunged from the monographs for a number of drugs for the first time. The intent was to set basic quality specifications to be met, but avoid explicit directions for formulation that might place unnecessary legal restrictions on how large-scale manufacture was to be carried out.[15]

Originally conceived as a formulary, the NF did not include uncombined botanical drugs and medicinal chemicals ("simples") until the Fourth Edition (1916). This change of character was limited to simples that entered into a compound formula elsewhere in the NF and was stimulated by the new obligations implied by official status. To one writer in 1912 it would seem more logical if "Our Pharmacopoeia should embody simple substances alone," and transfer compound chemical and galenical preparations to the NF, where they would fit neatly into the original formulary concept.[16] Out of step with the trend, it was an idea that could not be taken seriously, especially given the traditional concept of USP scope.

The number of substances and compositions for which specifications were set by each of the twelve NF editions within the scope of this paper (1896–1970) ranged from 454 to 1009. The number of admissions and deletions in each revision cycle could be affected somewhat by USP decisions on admissions, which took priority as a matter of policy. Thus it could happen that a monograph carefully worked up by the NF Committee for a newly admitted drug could be preempted for use in the next USP. Conversely, many monographs deleted from the USP often could be taken over verbatim into the NF—especially after the structure of specifications in NF monographs came to correspond so closely with those of the USP.

If we compare the net number of substances and compositions recognized in each edition, as shown in **Table I**, it becomes apparent that there was no rigid preconception about what the size of the NF should be. About two-thirds of the dramatic increase between the 1906 and 1916 editions reflects recognition of uncompounded botanical and chemical ingredients for the first time. Other influences stemming from the 1906 Food and Drugs Act may account for at least part of the remainder. Between the 1916 and 1965 editions, the net admissions fluctuated within a narrow range of about 20%. A striking increase during the revision cycle between 1965 and 1970 can be attributed largely to the government's retrospective review of the therapeutic efficacy of prescription drugs on the market and to the NF's own shift toward therapeutic efficacy as a criterion for admissions. There were 221 articles dropped from the new edition (NF XIII), and nearly twice that number were newly admitted, an unprecedented 41% of the total. The newly recognized drugs rep-

TABLE I: CHANGE IN NUMBER OF NF DRUGS (SIMPLE AND COMPOSITE)

Edition	Date	Total*
I	1880	435
II	1896	784
III	1906	486
IV	1916	784
V	1926	762
VI	1936	689
VII	1942	732
VIII	1947	818
IX	1950	717
X	1955	733
XI	1960	c. 830
XII	1965	783
XIII	1970	992
XIV	1975	1009

*Totals are taken from prefatory material in each edition except NF VIII, which was tabulated from personal count. Certain totals before NF IX (1950) may include the descriptive general chapters for monographs on an individual class of preparation (e.g., fluid extracts), an upward variance of not more than 3%.

resented a broad range of therapeutic classes, such as various oral contraceptives, the first prophylactic anti-viral product, cardiac drugs, new diagnostic aids, hypoglycemics, tranquilizers, an array of potent steroids, and the first aerosol propellants.[17]

An early question of admissions policy arose from an issue that agitated American pharmacists during the late nineteenth century. Mass production and mass promotion of prefabricated proprietary remedies were cutting into the small-scale manufacture and prescription compounding that traditionally had been a central role of the practicing pharmacist. One motivation among pharmacists for supporting the youthful NF was, as one pharmacist expressed it, "to rid them or at least offer some relief of the existing [proprietary] evil."[18] Pharmacists felt that the public interest was on their side, since even prescription proprietaries often were promoted in a misleading manner, were at least partly secret in composition, and were tradenamed in a fanciful way that required pharmacists to stock several different brands of what often turned out to be essentially the same drug. It was a losing battle, but one that the more professionally conscious pharmacists waged well into the present century. One resource to use in the struggle was the *National Formulary*, whose formulas could provide prescribing physicians with remedies comparable to the proprietaries, but were of known composition, rationally named and represented, and locally produced.[19] The NF always abided by a policy that no monograph would be included for a drug "under the proprietary or trade-mark name, or if the composition or process of manufacture is secret." Moreover, it was wary of seeming to offer imitations of the proprietaries then taking physicians and the public by storm.[20] But after NF I, the subsequent editions offered some formulas of this character.[21] Although proprietary manufacturers expressed concern, the respected pharmacist Martin I. Wilbert responded that "the preparations of which the N.F. preparations are said to be imitations are themselves not original and have nothing to be imitated . . . "[22]

Unease also surfaced occasionally because the NF "does not assume any responsibility for the therapeutic value of any preparation," a statement conscientiously inserted in each edition, at least from NF IV (1916) onward. A common argument in support of the policy was that a physician or patient has a right to expect a drug of well defined and uniform quality pharmaceutically even when experts consider the drug not particularly good therapeutically.

The conceptual difference between the NF and the USP concerning therapeutic efficacy might have narrowed sooner if a move following passage of the 1906 Act had succeeded. The NF Committee sought "the cooperation of the medical profession and the Medical Departments of the National Government;" but this effort misfired within two years when "it quickly developed that the medical interest in the [NF] work was entirely therapeutic, while the basis of revision was directed to be pharmaceutic."[23] Thereafter one or more prominent physicians contributed to revision work, but only when invited and mainly to help estimate the *extent* of medical usage of a drug, when deciding questions of admission.

The question surfaced again a few years later when the pharmacy dean at the University of Iowa wrote, "My thought is that the only reason why medicinal substances should be given recognition by the NF is because of their positive and unquestioned therapeutic value. The NF will not be scientifically sound, considering the purpose for which it is created, until this is true."[24] Other voices in 1920 spoke to the same point. Rufus A. Lyman, M.D., of Nebraska agreed that the current policy "tends to promote and prolong the polypharmacy of former ages. . . . Certainly, the common usage of a drug or a formula is no justification," he contended, "for making a standard for it in the N.F." An industrial scientist agreed, but a well-known practitioner in Brooklyn waved a slogan: "What physicians prescribe, we pharmacists shall prepare!"[25]

The conservative voices prevailed until a quarter century later, when a different Chairman, Justin L. Powers, alerted readers to a fundamental change in a back-handed way by saying, "The admission of drugs to this edition has, as in the past, been based not only on therapeutic value, but also upon the extent of use."[26] NF X (1955) went a step further by announcing that, while extent of use remained a criterion, "Therapeutic value, as a criterion for admission to N.F. X, was given greater priority than heretofore by the Committee on

National Formulary in reaching final decisions on scope."[27] In the following revision the phrase "greater priority" has been supplanted by a statement that "The admission of drugs to this edition has been based *mainly* on therapeutic value as determined by an Advisory Committee on Admissions."[28] Finally, in 1961 the NF Board (the erstwhile NF Committee) approved a policy that "drugs are admitted *only* on the basis of their recognized therapeutic value."[29] That the issue had not been laid entirely to rest is implied by a statement in the NF XIII (1970): "The National Formulary Board unanimously and emphatically reaffirmed the policy adopted in 1961 and initially employed for NF XII—namely, that therapeutic value would serve as the sole criterion in considering articles to be admitted to the National Formulary for medicinal purposes."[30] Thus a final step had been taken in bringing the operational policies and program into close alignment with the USP.

The dosage forms utilized to convey medicaments to the patient likewise contributed importantly, if less controversially, to the NF's changing character. An impression of how NF dosage forms evolved quantitatively can be gained from **Table II**, which shows the approximate number of monographs for each form of administration at the founding, at the time of merger with the USP, and at midpoint in the NF's history as a separate standard-setting agency.[31] The changing forms of medicaments specified by the NF and USP have been portrayed most vividly (up to 1945) through an array of graphs published by Osborne and Lee.[32]

When we recall that the original NF was a classic formulary of mainly polypharmacal combinations, it underscores how radical was the change of character when we read in the 1970 edition: "The [NF] Board also defined its policy with regard to admission of drug combinations—namely that the NF monographs for combination dosage forms will be limited to those combinations for which there is a therapeutic advantage to the patient as contrasted with administration of the separate individual therapeutically-active ingredients."[33] A centuries-long tradition was ending, when pharmacists took pride in their ability to combine multiple drugs into a single medicament, thus obviating the need for a patient to take several separate medicaments. The potency of many modern medicaments argued against the old practice of locking in fixed dosages of several active substances by combining them as a single drug product.

Face and Format of the NF

The NF's structure and means for conveying quality standards have been part of its changing character. A few examples will be sufficient to give an impression of the evolving format.

After the book became official, it steadily took on the colorations of the USP. As early as 1910 there were suggestions, as Lyman

TABLE II: NUMBER OF PRODUCTS IN EACH NF DOSAGE FORM

	1888 N.F. I	1926 N.F. V	1970 N.F. XIII
Aerosols	0	0	6
Ampuls	0	7	1
Capsules	0	0	45
Cement	0	0	1
Confections	0	2	0
Creams	0	0	13
Dressings	0	1	0
Elixirs	86	65	14
Emulsions	11	5	1
Extracts	2	13	2
Fluidextracts	51	104	4
Gels and Jellies	0	0	2
General Monographs	2	15	29
Glycerites	7	5	1
Infusions	2	4	0
Injections	0	0	102
Liniments and Dentiliments	8	12	0
Lotions	4	7	6
Magmas and Milks	1	3	3
Miscellaneous	54	75	0
Mixtures	19	13	1
Ointments and Mulls	5	23	20
Papers	0	1	0
Pastes	0	7	1
Pellets	0	0	3
Pencils, Medicinal	0	1	0
Petroxolins	0	17	0
Pills	27	23	1
Plasters	4	2	0
Powders	15	14	4
Salts, Effervescent	10	9	1
Solutions	41	37	39
Spirits	12	11	3
Sprays	0	5	0
Suppositories	0	1	9
Suspensions	0	0	31
Syrups	35	37	21
Tablets	0	7	189
Tinctures	32	55	6
Troches	0	2	0
Waters	4	2	3
Wines	12	0	0
Total of Dosage Forms	444	585	562
Total Drugs and Chemicals	0	214	460

Kebler of the USDA Bureau of Chemistry put it, "that ways and means be brought about where the two Committees [NF and USP] act jointly for the purpose of improving both books."[34] Within a decade it could be claimed that such coordination between the NF and USP had "made it possible to maintain strict harmony in the style of treatment and also to avoid duplicating titles, and establishing two standards for the same article."[35]

This circumstance led some to the idea of actual merger. A wholesale druggist had suggested in 1908 a single book of drug standards, embodying both the NF and the USP. The APhA President recommended, two years later, that a committee "consider the desirability and practicability of the publication of the National Formulary by the United States Pharmacopoeial Convention."[36] One pharmacy dean noted in 1920 that the NF "now has the appearance of a second pharmacopoeia" and wondered "why the N.F. should be kept within the A.Ph.A. control."[37]

In NF IV (1916) for the first time, the Committee had to deal with the individual botanical and chemical substances (e.g., Cascarilla or Precipitated Calcium Phosphate) that were ingredients of formulas for which the USP had not set standards. Such substances were listed in a new Part II (97 pp.); but it seemed so awkward to have the simples and the composites listed separately, in two alphabets, that they were merged from 1936 onward into a single alphabet. The same fate had befallen a separate A-to-Z section in NF III (1906) into which the formulas deleted from the previous USP had been swept so that standards would continue to be maintained. With the next edition the transfers from the USP were absorbed into the NF proper.

An enduring feature introduced into NF V (1926), and the concurrent USP, was the practice of placing at the end of each monograph for a simple botanical or chemical a list of all preparations into which it entered as an essential ingredient.

After the FDC Act of 1938 identified as "drugs" the substances intended for the diagnosis of disease, the NF organized a panel of about ninety experts in that field. Their evaluations resulted in a new chapter on diagnostic substances, beginning with NF VII.[38]

At first the NF monographs did not include an expression of dosage, probably to avoid any implication of encouraging over-the-counter prescribing by pharmacists. However, this feature would have obvious utility in the proper practice of both medicine and pharmacy; so for each internal medication in NF III (1906) an "average" dose was expressed in both the metric and the apothecary systems of metrology, and from NF XI (1960) onward in the metric system alone. Uneasiness with the term "average dose" led to what was called the "usual dose," and eventually in many monographs to a "usual dose range" (NF XIII, 1970). As a further aid to students and practitioners, NF X (1955) and USP XV (1955) introduced a

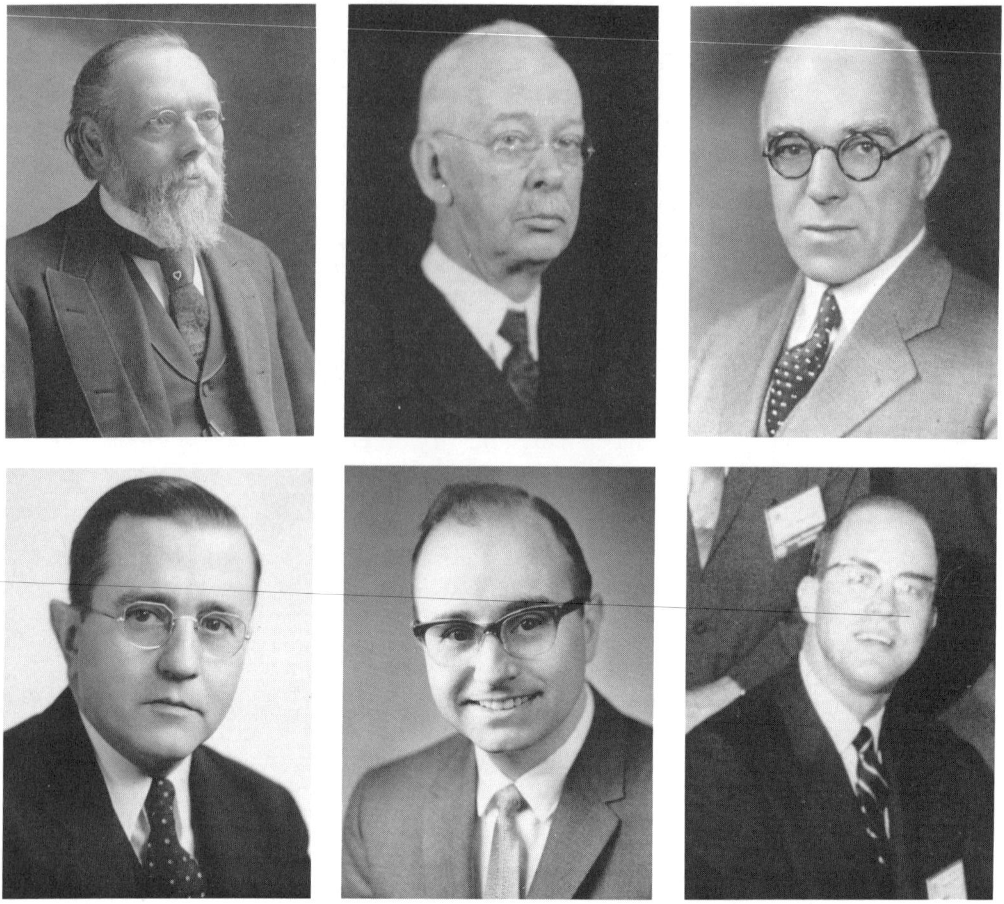

Six chairmen directed revisions of the National Formulary during the period discussed in this paper (l. to r.): C. Lewis Diehl (1889–1917; NF II, III, IV), Wilbur L. Scoville (1919–29; NF V), Edmund N. Gathercoal (1930–40; NF VI), Justin L. Powers (1940–60; NF VII, VIII, IX, X, XI), Edward G. Feldmann (1960–69; NF XII, XIII), John V. Bergen (1970–74; NF XIV). (Photos courtesy of the APhA and Kremers Reference Files, University of Wisconsin-Madison.)

statement of the best-known pharmacologic action of each medicament, while disclaiming intent or authority to circumscribe the actual range of use in practice.[39]

A section of "Special Notices," first introduced in NF IV (1916), became increasingly important because it included "the basic guidelines for the interpretation and application of the standards, tests, assays, and other specifications of the National Formulary, and obviate[d] the need to repeat throughout the book those definitions, interpretations or requirements that are pertinent."[40]

On the question of nomenclature, it seemed clear to the initial NF Committee that a self-respecting work would opt for Latinized drug names, conforming to a precedent set by the USP and by a vestige of the centuries-old tradition that recognized Latin as common coin of communication among the health professions internationally. The founders "selected what appeared to them the most suitable and expressive titles . . . " though they conceded that many "will never be ordered [by physicians] under their Latin names."[41] Unpersuaded, one prominent pharmacist claimed, "The use of names, too scientific and extended in their character, was a mistake, as the physicians did not understand them and would not make use of them in prescribing."[42] That especially perplexed pharmacists who looked to the NF to help counter the catchy and more memorable tradenames that industrialists assigned to the rising tide of proprietary drugs. Physicians increasingly wrote prescriptions for them rather than for the more complex "generic" titles of NF (and USP) medicaments–such as Elixir Ammonii Valerianatis et Quininae, or Emulsum Olei Morrhuae cum Calcii et Sodii Phosphatibus. The NF Committee got the message, tried to cope with it in revisions for NF III, and failed. Concluding that snappy titles were incompatible with sound principles of drug nomenclature, they reported to practitioners in the Preface: "In accordance with the expressed desire, an attempt was made to devise short synonyms or abbreviated titles for some of the lengthy ones now in use; but this virtually remained an attempt, having been found practicable only in a few instances."

The policy continued to be, "That [drug] nomenclature, titles, and synonyms be in conformity with the USP or with modern ideas, and that the titles should be descriptive of composition, and therapeutic or anatomical titles should be discouraged." One step in the desired direction was the devising of a standard abbreviation for the official title of each drug, "as an aid to prescription writing and for concise labelling."[43]

There had been portents from the beginning of another minor but notable change: dropping the sequential numbers that had been attached to the formulas of NF medicaments to simplify prescribing. The NF Committee apparently had not foreseen the complication of numerous future additions and deletions in the numbered series. Consequently, the number on a formula in the Second Edition might no longer be attached to the same formula as in the First Edition. One critic felt that some risk that a patient might receive the wrong medication did exist, and observed: "Of course it may be argued that no one should prescribe or order a medicinal preparation simply by an arbitrary number, but we also know that this is largely done, and will continue to be done."[44] With NF III (1906) the numbering of formulas was quietly and permanently abandoned.

By the end of World War II chemotherapy was ascendant; and stretching Latin nomenclature to label the products of modern pharmaco-medical science seemed to many an anachronism. For older practitioners there was a touch of sacrilege in the idea of downgrading the resounding Latinic phrases, one hallmark after all of a properly learned physician or pharmacist. Moreover, it was unseemly that patients should be worried with knowledge of the drugs in their regimen, which would be conveyed by prescribing in English. A compromise was reached in NF VIII (1947) when English titles became the primary nomenclature of the NF, and Latin titles were relegated to second place.[45] By NF X (1955) the Latin titles had been reduced to 8-point type alongside English-language common names (synonyms), and thereafter disappeared altogether, as they did also from the USP.

Structural formulas had been part of the nomenclature of pharmaceutical science and became increasingly common as a part of NF monographs during the 1940s. Sometimes a structural formula could even serve as the official definition of a drug, for example, naturally-occurring products for which an assay could not be devised. In the early 1960s the NF Committee undertook to rework the structural formulas for NF organic medicinals systematically, based on nuclei drawn in the style adopted by the International Union of Pure and Applied Chemistry. This, together with a reworking of the verbal chemical names, permitted NF XII (1965) to represent medicinal chemicals in a more uniform manner and to make the relationships among various drugs more apparent.

About this time the NF and USP had become more concerned about drug names in general, especially as hearings held by Senator Kefauver's committee sensitized government agencies, the professions, and the public, to the complexities of drug nomenclature, proprietary and nonproprietary—and to the impediment this offered to what came to be called "generic" prescribing. The ensuing Congressional "Drug Amendments of 1962" prohibited the official compendia from including more than one name for any drug; and that should be a simple and useful name. Consequently, the NF (like the USP) eliminated all synonyms from the monographs and reformed numerous drug titles in NF XII (1965).

This experience pointed up the need for selecting a simple and useful nonproprietary name early in the life of each drug. So an improved nomenclature program was launched in 1964 under the co-sponsorship of the American Pharmaceutical Association (as publisher of the NF), the American Medical Association, and the United States Pharmacopeia. Each sponsor was henceforth represented on the Council of United States Adopted Names, which selects an appropriate nonproprietary ("USAN") name for a new drug before it is considered for admission to the NF (or the USP).[46] While by no means a revolutionary change in NF character, it was a reform that pruned considerable verbal overgrowth from the thicket of drug nomenclature, as the appearance of NF XIII (1970) demonstrated.

Weights and measures and their accurate use have always been a special concern of pharmacists, by the nature of their work. An idea of the first NF Committee therefore soon came under careful scrutiny, namely that formulas "need not all be forced into one rigid, immutable, and uniform system of weights or of measures."[47] This initial mixed metrology seemed to increase the chance of error; moreover, it was out of joint with the USP of 1890, which had converted to the metric system. The NF II (1896) followed suit, quantifying formulas only in the metric system. It was a bold move not readily accepted.

One reviewer maintained that "a very large number of pharmacists have no metric weights and measures," and maintained that the work habits of physicians and pharmacists argue for showing equivalents in the apothecaries' system as a secondary option for prescription practice.[48] In contrast, one writer in *The Western Druggist* applauded the NF's decisiveness in the "overthrow of the antiquated, barbarous and mongrel systems of weights and measures still in vogue among the English-speaking nations." But metric did not yet have wide support among Americans, and physicians and pharmacists were no exception. They had a sentimental attachment to the apothecaries' system, which seemed peculiarly their own.[49]

Faced with marked resistance to change, the NF Committee backed off, and in the Third Edition (1906) presented all formulas in *both* systems, expressing a hope that this would "add to the utility and popularity of the *Formulary*." The master pharmacist M. I. Wilbert of Philadelphia apparently spoke for others when he termed the double system of weights and measures "one of the most unfortunate features" of the new NF.[50] While adoption of the metric system would continue to agitate discussion in America, the NF Committee made its final response in the next edition (NF IV, 1916) by reverting to the use of metric alone—except for retaining the apothecaries system as a secondary expression of average doses.

The Changing Purpose of the NF

Looking back on the constellation of events, we see sweeping changes in the character of the *National Formulary* during the eighty-seven years from first publication that it remained under the sponsorship of the American Pharmaceutical Association.[51] Underpinning the character and degree of these changes were especially four influences: new expectations and responsibilities evolving out of an unexpected official status, accelerating progress in the pharmaceutical science and technology on which standard-setting depends, the industrialization of drug making, and the U.S. Pharmacopeia as the acknowledged bellwether for the National Formulary. The combined impact dramatically altered the book.

Though the NF no longer held much practical utility for even the best-educated community pharmacists, it is well to recall that pharmacists continued to supply a public service through the National Formulary—by sponsorship of this complex endeavor through their national professional society, by their volunteer service on NF Committees and subcommittees, and by crucial support of NF operations through their perennial purchase of a book that served an ideal. It was an American ideal that strikes a balance of responsibility among the private sector of health sciences, the government, and the pharmaceutical industry, for the purpose of assuring pharmaceutical supplies of predictably high quality.

It was an ideal shared by the *Pharmacopeia of the United States.* Indeed, after 1960 conceptual differences between the NF and USP were slight. This invited serious questioning about the need for two standard-setting agencies, the need for two "pharmacopeias" in the United States. How that question was answered would soon open a new phase in the history[52] of setting standards for the nation's drug supply.

Notes and References

1. It should be noted, bibliographically, that the term "Unofficinal" was altered to "Unofficial" in the title of the Second Edition. Thereafter, the title was simply *The National Formulary.* The name of the American Pharmaceutical Association (APhA hereafter) always appeared on the title page as publisher; but a place of publication was not designated until the Sixth Edition indicated Washington, D. C., where the Association had opened its headquarters building in 1934. This paper follows accepted usage in employing a Roman numeral to identify a particular *edition* of NF (whereas the convention is to use a Roman numeral to identify a particular *revision* of the *Pharmacopoeia of the United States of America*). The diphthong was dropped from the spelling of "Pharmacopeia" in the Fourteenth Revision (1950); and this modernized spelling is used in this paper, except for quotations, for the sake of uniformity. The *date* cited for each NF edition refers to the year of publication for the first four editions; thereafter it refers to the year in which the edition became *official*, as shown on the title page.
2. Glenn Sonnedecker and George Urdang. "Legalization of Drug Standards Under State Laws in the United States of America," *Food Drug Cosmetic Law Journal* 8 (1953): 749. The definition of what constitutes a "pharmacopeia" in a modern sense has been a matter of discussion. A certain nongovernmental authority to foster uniformity of medicaments (as held by the USP before 1906) has antecedents in some of the early European drug books, such as the *Nuovo Receptario* of 1498 for the city-state of Florence. (See Martin Levey, "The Italian Phar-

macopoeia and the Influence of Arabic Pharmacy," *Pharmacy in History* 12 (1970): 13.) Even after becoming "official" under Federal law, the NF and USP could be enforced nationally only in what courts defined as *inter*state commerce. This limitation motivated individual states to adopt parallel statutes that could enforce drug standards in *intra*state commerce.

3. NF IV (1919), x, and Henry P. Hynson, "The National Formulary; Its Future and Some Attending Responsibilities," *Midland Druggist and Pharmaceutical Review* 44 (1910): 482.
4. Lyman F. Kebler to James H. Beal, 12 September 1940 and Beal to Kebler, 19 September 1940; transcripts in folder "A2:Beal, J.H.," in Kremers Reference Files, F. B. Power Pharmaceutical Library, University of Wisconsin. George Urdang and Glenn Sonnedecker, "Authoritative English-Language Drug Compendia Supplementing Pharmacopoeias," *Food Drug Cosmetic Law Journal* 8 (1953): 486 and 494.
5. "A.Ph.A. Sustains National Formulary as Standard," *Pharmaceutical Era* 42 (1909): 231 and P. Henry Utech, "The NF V," *Journal of the American Pharmaceutical Association* 10 (1921): 275.
6. The 1938 law required that compliance with official specifications be demonstrated by the *procedure* stated in the NF and USP. This increased the importance of the test methods, as distinguished from the quantitative and qualitative specifications. Other symptoms of intensified responsibility included changing the APhA bylaws (1967) to enhance the legal foundation of the NF; renaming the Committee on National Formulary as the National Formulary Board (NF XIV, 1975, xliv); and broadening the title and scope of the *Bulletin of the National Formulary Committee* (f. 1930) as *Drug Standards* from 1951 on.
7. Lyman F. Kebler, "Report of Committee on What the National Formulary Should Be," *Midland Drugg. and Pharmaceu. Rev.* 44 (1910): 27. This was a special committee of the Washington, DC, branch of the APhA.
8. Examples of NF studies in progress at that time included: developing a test for ampul glass; designing a system of nomenclature for precise color specifications; quantifying better the moisture present in medicinal chemicals; improving the method for determining the volatile-oil content of crude drugs; and checking the adequacy of NF methods for preventing deterioration of pepsin products once they leave the production laboratory. E. N. Gathercoal, "Report on the National Formulary Research Projects of 1936," *Bulletin of the National Formulary Committee* 22 March 1937, 2548–2554.
9. E. F. K[elly], "National Formulary Revision," *J. Am. Pharm. Assoc.,* 28 (1939): 630. Beginning in 1962 the American Medical Association and The United States Pharmacopeial Convention became co-sponsors of the Drug Standards Laboratory. In 1975 the Laboratory was transferred to the headquarters of the U.S. Pharmacopeia in Bethesda, Md.
10. NF XII (1965), xvi.
11. NF XIII (1970), xxvii.
12. Hynson, "National Formulary," (n. 3), p. 484. The respected Professor Edward Kremers from Wisconsin also felt strongly: "It is altogether wrong to regard the N.F. as [merely] a lumber chamber for the U.S.P." Kremers to A. L. Buzzell, folder "C32(d)I:USA," F. B. Power Pharmaceutical Library, University of Wisconsin.

13. Wilbur L. Scoville, "The National Formulary," *J. Am. Pharm. Assoc.* 10 (1921): 245; see also Henry Kraemer, "What Should be the Scope of the Next NF," *Bulletin of Pharmacy* 34 (March 1920): 34.
14. Hynson, "National Formulary," (n.3), p. 485.
15. NF VI (1936), 493. It testified to how deeply the tradition of small-scale manufacture persisted among some pharmacists when—as the NF became more self-consciously official and scientific, and the number of quantitative formulas began to dwindle—the APhA launched (1929) a *Pharmaceutical Recipe Book* consisting of hundreds of unofficial formulas for homely remedies and household products. See Glenn Sonnedecker (rev.), *Kremers and Urdang's History of Pharmacy,* 4th ed. (Philadelphia, 1976), 281.
16. John Roemer, "The National Formulary in the making," *Merck's Report* 21 (1912): 208.
17. NF XIII (1970), xxi. For a detailed picture of the individual drugs and the length of time they were recognized during the first half century of the NF, consult H. A. Langenhan, "A Half Century of the National Formulary 1880–1930," *J. Am. Pharm. Assoc.* 15 (1926), Nos. 8–12 and 16 (1927), Nos. 1–6; also collated as a separate booklet (n. p., n. d., 99 pp.). Part I of this painstaking work shows the primary titles of all preparations A-to-Z (also the English titles and synonyms) and the editions in which each preparation appeared. Part II does the same for the simple botanical and chemical ingredients, A-to-Z. For admissions and deletions, 1930 to 1970, see the unpublished card index compiled by George D. Beal, Kremers Reference Files, F. B. Power Pharmaceutical Library, University of Wisconsin–Madison. Although admissions and deletions always had been based on the presumed extent of use of a drug, the revision for NF VI (1936) may be the first that quantified extent of use through field surveys of actual prescription records, a technique too demanding to be sustained in subsequent decades. See Edmund N. Gathercoal, ed., *The Prescription Ingredient Survey* (n. p., APhA, 1933). The frequency threshold for admission (with few exceptions) was that a substance must be used in at least 20% of American drugstores or occur as an ingredient at least once in each 10,000 prescriptions. A more limited field survey guided the extensive deletions (especially botanical drugs) and additions reflected in NF IX (1950). See *Bull. Natl. Form. Comm.* 15 (1947): 137.
18. F. Hemm, "A Few Remarks on the National Formulary," *Druggists Circular* 35 (1891): 201.
19. Howard C. Newton, "Address of the Chairman," Section on Practical Pharmacy, *J. Am. Pharm. Assoc.* 15 (1926): 1129.
20. NF V (1926), xiv.
21. C. Lewis Diehl, "The National Formulary; Its Attitude to Pharmaceutical Proprietaries," *Journal of the American Medical Association* 47 (1906): 1826; pp. 6f. of reprint.
22. Martin I. Wilbert, "The National Formulary and Proprietary Remedies," *Pharmaceu. Era,* 46 (1913) 547. Discussion of this issue in the pharmaceutical press peaked during the first quarter of this century. Some other examples are by A. Weinstein, *Druggists' Circular and Chemical Gazette* 49 (1905): 322; E. Spease, *Bull. Pharm.* 34 (1920): 239; F. Hemm, *Pharmaceutical Record* 12 (1891): 102; C. Lewis Diehl, *Proceedings of the American Pharaceutical Association* 43 (1895): 53,

and Sidney Rauschenberg, *American Druggist and Pharmaceutical Record* 28 (1896): 366. A similar motivation was involved in founding the *National Formulary* of Great Britain, which produced better results in reducing the use of unoriginal specialties in medical care, apparently because of a linkage to prescribing under Britain's national health insurance. *Journal Mondial de Pharmacie* (1960), No. 1: 17.

23. NF IV (1916), xi.
24. R. A. Kuever, "What Should Be the Scope of the Next NF," *Bull. Pharm.* 34 (1920): 99.
25. *Bull. Pharm.* 34 (1920): Rufus A. Lyman, 141, Oliver A. Farwell, 189, and Otto Raubenheimer, 140.
26. NF VIII (1947), x.
27. NF X (1955), xiv.
28. NF XI (1960), ix. This new Advisory Committee consisted of expert physicians, with the exception of three key staff members of the NF and USP.
29. "The National Formulary," multilith 8.5 × 11″, from The National Formulary, Washington, D.C., dated 1 June 1967, p. 1, folder "C32(d)I: USA", Kremers Reference Files, F. B. Power Pharmaceutical Library, University of Wisconsin-Madison. Italics added.
30. NF XIII (1970), xxi.
31. Data for editions I (1888) and V (1926) are mainly from a tabulation published in NF VI (1936), 494, although some adjustments have been made (because of questions of terminology or interpretation). Whether or not a compound preparation should be treated as a separate dosage form is not always obvious and probably led to some inconsistencies of classification.
32. George E. Osborne and C. O. Lee, "Graphic Story of Official Galenicals," *Bull. Natl. Form. Comm.* 15 (1947): 185–204.
33. NF XIII (1970), xxi.
34. Lyman F. Kebler, "Report of Committee on What the NF Should Be" [D.C. branch, APhA], *Midland Drugg. and Pharm. Rev.* 44 (1910): 26.
35. E. Fullerton Cook, "Fourth Edition of the National Formulary," *Drugg. Circ.* 60 (1916): 541. Cook observed that the NF is "an auxiliary to, not a rival of the Pharmacopoeia."
36. Jacob Weil in *Proceedings of the National Wholesale Druggists Association* 1908, 287; Henry H. Rusby, "President's Address," *Proc. Am. Pharm. Assoc.* 58 (1910), 442. The committee later replied: "The recommendation of our honored President is not approved." (*Proc.*, 483).
37. Ernest R. Jones, "What should be the Scope of the Next National Formulary," *Bull. Pharm.* 34 (1920): 100.
38. E. F. Kelly, "National Formulary Revision," *J. Am. Pharm. Assoc.* 28 (1939): 630.
39. NF X (1955), xvi and 8.
40. The central office for the NF once claimed that "at least two-thirds of the inquiries" it received could have been answered by correspondents themselves if they had studied the General Notices and Requirements, as the section was then called (NF XIV, 1975, xxi). Not to be confused with the statement of "General Principles," which were reformulated for each successive revision period, to serve as guidelines for collaborators across the country in generating the next NF edition. A section introduced in NF IV (1916), "Special Tests and Reagents," provided

general tests—for example to determine heavy-metal contaminations, or the amount of fiber in crude drugs—but it was replaced after NF V by giving appropriate cross-references to tests in the USP.

41. NF I (1888), vi.
42. Albert Ebert, commenting on the "Report of the Committee on National Formulary," *Proc. Am. Pharm. Assoc.,* 52 (1904), 205.
43. NF IV (1916), xii and xv.
44. Anon., "The Number of National Formulary Preparations," *Pharmaceu. Era* 17 (1897): 743.
45. An invited historical article influenced considerably the argument in favor of abandoning pharmaceutical Latin: George Urdang, "The Place of Latin in the Official Standards of Pharmacy," *Bull. Natl. Form.* 12 (1944), Nos. 11 and 12: 201–220.
46. NF XII (1965), xvii.
47. NF I (1880), vi.
48. "New Books," *Merck's Report,* 5 (1896): 251.
49. The metric system already had won the day in pharmaceutical science, but encountered slower acceptance in medical care. See Gregory J. Higby and Glenn Sonnedecker, "Adoption of the Metric System by the U.S. Pharmacopeia," *Journal of the History of Medicine and Allied Sciences* 40 (1985): 207–213.
50. M. I. Wilbert, "The Scope and the Shortcomings of the National Formulary," *American Journal of Pharmacy* 79 (1907): 210. See also "Editorial Comment," *Drugg. Circ.* 51 (1907): 760.
51. Much of the change and its timing has been response to leadership provided by the Chairmen of the Committee (later, Board) on National Formulary. Their names, the editions for which they were responsible, and years in office are: Charles Rice, I (1883–1888); C. Lewis Diehl, II, III, IV (1889–1917); Wilbur L. Scoville, V (1919–1929); Edmund N. Gathercoal, VI (1930–1940); Justin L. Powers, VII, VIII, IX, X, XI (1940–1960); Edward G. Feldmann, XII, XIII (1961–1969); John V. Bergen, XIV (1970–1974).
52. On the history of the National Formulary, heretofore only a few essays have appeared, such as: C. Lewis Diehl, "The Evolution of the National Formulary," *Bulletin of the American Pharmaceutical Association* 4 (1909): 14–18 and 44–47; Justin L. Powers, "History, Significance and Future of the National Formulary," *Food Drug Cosmetic Law Quarterly* 1 (1946): 577–587; Justin L. Powers, "Drug Standards in the United States," I and II, in: *The Pharmaceutical Sciences; Third Annual Visiting Lecture Series* (Austin, 1960), 231–250; Glenn Sonnedecker, "Drug Standards Become Official," in: *The Early Years of Federal Food and Drug Control* (Madison, 1982), 28–39; anon., "Highlights on National Formulary History," *Drugg. Circ.* 74 (July 1930): 16 and 58; and the historical summary in each edition of the NF.

The NF-USP Merger: Controversies and Consequences

by Edward G. Feldmann

During the past few years, the business world and the financial community have witnessed a plethora of corporate mergers, leveraged buy-outs, corporate acquisitions, hostile or friendly takeovers, and various other types of similar activities. However, back in the late 1960s and early 1970s such events were a relative rarity. Consequently, the NF-USP consolidation, which occurred officially on January 2, 1975, was a fore-runner to such activities that are now rather commonplace in the business field. Moreover, in its day, it was an event that was as controversial, as fiercely negotiated, and as intensely emotional as any of the headline grabbing corporate mergers that have been waged in recent years. Indeed, beyond the simple economic considerations that are the essential basis for the vast majority of corporate mergers, there were assorted professional, scientific, legislative, and technical considerations involved with the NF-USP merger proposal that introduced several additional important dimensions.

This "compendial marriage" ranks as one of the most significant events in the history of the U.S. official compendia, of drug standardization in the United States, and of the worldwide concept of drug quality. The people charged with guiding the fortunes and shaping the future of the USP and NF were highly conscious of the enormous obligations they had to the health professions, to their respective constituencies, and to society in general, with respect to ascertaining the best direction to proceed and then to do all that they could to move effectively toward that common objective. On this basis, a brief examination of the circumstances leading up to the merger, the pro and con arguments surrounding such a proposed merger, the negotiations involved, and the subsequent events to accomplish the merger is essential to any review of the National Formulary's history. Furthermore, collectively, these events and activities constitute a very interesting story in the broad panorama of American pharmacy and the quest for high quality drug standards.

Why an NF?

Before we consider NF-USP merger, it is important to review why the NF came into being in the first place. In preparing my remarks, I was aware that Gregory Higby would be discussing the founding of the National Formulary. Therefore, I will be brief on the subject of "Why an NF?" However, it is important to emphasize several points, as follows:

(a) The USP of the 1870s and early 1880s was very selective in the articles that it recognized for inclusion.
(b) Drugs and medicines of that era were chemically crude, and of dubious effectiveness by current standards.
(c) There was virtually no drug industry in the modern sense of the term and almost all dispensed products were compounded by the pharmacist (or physician) in the local pharmacy or medical office.
(d) There was no product standardization except for the drug monographs appearing in the then-current USP. Specifically, there was no FDA; there was no Federal Food, Drug, and Cosmetic Act; there were none of the many other state and federal laws, controls, and monitoring agencies that we take for granted today.

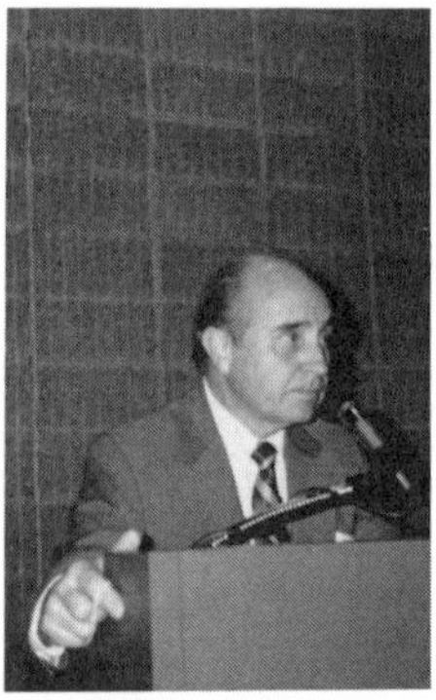

Edward G. Feldmann, Ph.D., *is President of Pharmaceutical Consultant Services of Falls Church, Virginia. From 1960–1970 he was Director and Chairman of the National Formulary. In addition he had general supervisory responsibility for the National Formulary from 1960–1975, and for the Drug Standards Laboratory from 1959–1975. Between 1959 and 1985 Dr. Feldmann was the principal scientist on the APhA staff, serving as Vice President for Scientific Affairs, Executive Secretary of the Academy of Pharmaceutical Sciences, and Editor of the Journal of Pharmaceutical Sciences.*

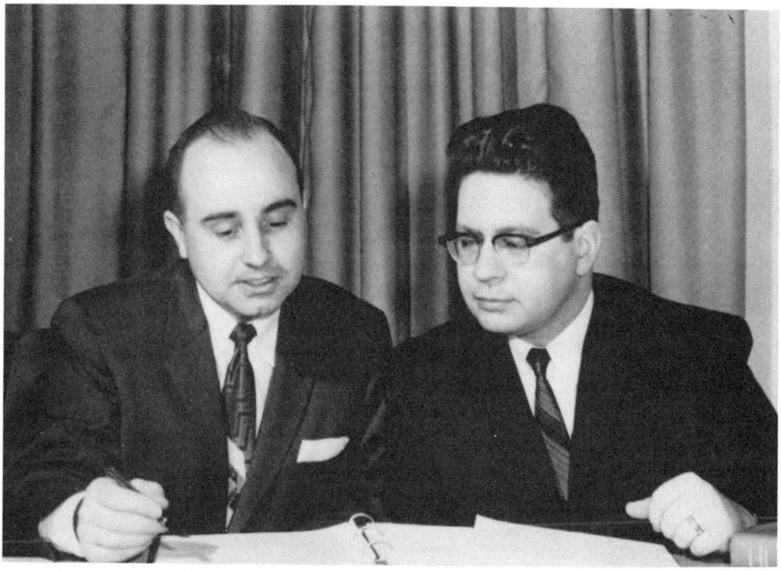

Figure 1. *A key event in the "modernization/revitalization" of the National Formulary was the establishment of the jointly sponsored Drug Standards Laboratory at the APhA Headquarters Building in late 1961. Pictured above, in January 1962, are NF Director Edward G. Feldmann (l.) and Jerome I. Bodin (r.), the newly appointed first Director of this restructured laboratory.*

Given these conditions, the NF of 1888 filled an important role in helping to standardize the nomenclature, composition, and quality of widely prescribed products. This all aside from any questions as to the inherent effectiveness or safety of the active ingredients contained in those products. This important role of the first NF continued for many years thereafter as identification and purity tests became more sophisticated, as assay procedures became more accurate and precise, and as the determination of product quality became more refined and defined.

Changing Conditions Affect the NF

Again, in preparing this paper, I was aware that Glenn Sonnedecker would be discussing the changing character of the NF. Hence, I will also be brief on this subject, but several points need to be emphasized in order to understand why the role of the NF in the mid-1970s had totally changed from that of the late 1880s. Similarly, by the late 1960s, the need for a separate, independent compendium of drug standards increasingly was being questioned due to changing circumstances.

First of all, the American pharmaceutical industry developed fully and became the source of 99% of dispensed drug products—a reversal of the situation in the mid-1880s. In the 1880s the NF served as a formulation guide (or "recipe book" if you will) for the pharmacist as to how to make the individually listed drug products, while by the 1970s, the NF no longer filled this function because dispensed products were all pre-compounded.

Second, drug laws were enacted at the federal and state level. These included the first Federal Pure Food and Drugs Act of 1906 and the current Federal Food, Drug, and Cosmetic Act of 1938. In addition, there have been major updates including the Drug Amendments of 1962. Respectively, these laws addressed drug adulteration and misbranding, proof of safety, and therapeutic effectiveness. Other laws prohibited dispensing various drugs without a prescription from a duly authorized prescriber, defined how drugs would be officially named, established procedures for new drug approval, regulated the advertising of drugs, and provided definitions that were essential to an orderly drug marketplace.

Third, the American Medical Association established operational units to review drug efficacy and relative efficacy, thereby relieving both the USP and the NF of their need to serve a primary role in those areas. The AMA Council on Pharmacy and Chemistry and its successor groups assumed a major responsibility in this general regard.

Fourth, a network of Federal, state, and local government laboratories and surveillance operations was established. It gradually filled the function of overseeing the performance of drug manufacturers, the quality of drug products, and all the related duties that FDA and other state and federal agencies now perform to ensure the quality of pharmaceutical products.

Fifth, the complexity of tests and standards grew beyond comprehension. In the 1880s the average neighborhood pharmacy was suitably equipped with simple reagents and chemical glassware to conduct all the laboratory procedures described in the NF or USP. However, by the 1970s compendial tests and assays commonly required the use of elaborate, highly sophisticated equipment costing millions of dollars and full-time, specially-trained technical personnel.

Sixth, the nature, composition, and duties of the cadre of volunteers serving on the compendial revision committees totally changed. In the 1880s, the NF revision committee consisted entirely of pharmacists engaged in full-time community practice who perhaps did some part-time teaching. In the case of the USP, the revision committee had just been opened to include pharmacy practitioners because, until then, it had been composed almost exclusively of practicing physicians. However, as the involvement and influence of the pharmaceutical industry and of the government developed,

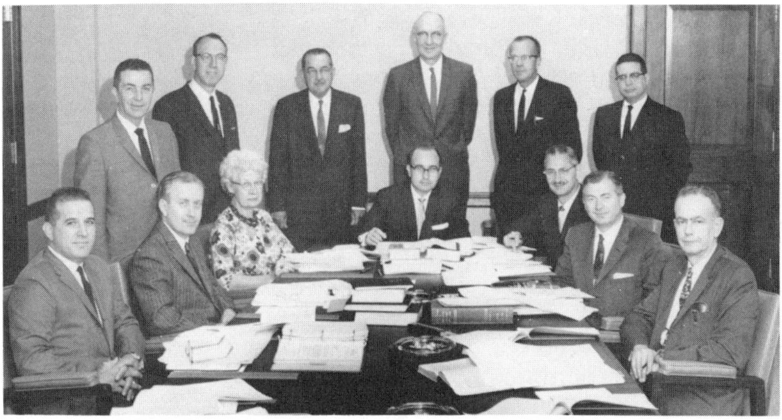

Figure 2. *The most dramatic changes in National Formulary scope, policy, and direction took place during the tenure of the 1960–1964 NF Board which was responsible for preparing NF XII. The overall impact of those changes brought the NF into a parallel position with the USP and made future merger a realistic possibility. Pictured above, in August 1962, are the members of that historic NF Board. Seated, l. to r., are J. A. Scigliano, H. F. Shirkey, B. Lyons (secretary to the NF Director), Board Chairman and NF Director E. G. Feldmann, S. W. Goldstein, E. Brochmann-Hanssen, and F. R. Franzoni; standing, l. to r., are F. A. Maurina, USP Director L. C. Miller (guest), H. H. Schaffer, C. L. Graham, E. O. Krueger, and Laboratory Director J. I. Bodin (guest). Absent was member B. Fortune.*

volunteer help was sought from these areas. However, the most crucial changes occurred in academia. Schools of pharmacy had supplied the backbone of volunteer support for the compendia during the first half of the twentieth Century. This began to shift by the early 1950s and, as academic volunteer support gradually dried up, the compendia experienced a serious short-fall of qualified volunteer assistance.

Separate Compendia Begin to be Questioned

When the National Formulary was first established in 1888, there was a clear distinction between it and the USP of that era. Specifically, the USP professed to restrict its coverage to a sort of "blue ribbon" list of drugs whose use and value had been most firmly established. There were, however, many other widely used drugs—some even more widely used than their USP counterparts—that were not in the USP and for which appropriate standardization was needed. Hence, "extent of use" became the original basic criterion for inclusion in the NF of non-USP articles.

The NF also served an important function by giving compendial recognition to valuable new drugs that had not yet achieved the track record of use which would qualify them for USP status. Finally, as newer drugs came along and supplanted the drugs that had been in the USP, it was felt that the NF should provide coverage to these still well-regarded and widely-used articles even though they no longer enjoyed top place in their class. This concept led NF officials during the early twentieth century to refer to the NF as "a stepping stone to, and from, USP recognition."

However, the various changes that were enumerated above served to diminish the early reasons for establishing the NF. In addition, the character and concepts of the USP itself were undergoing some similar, albeit less dramatic changes. The composite result was a blurring of distinction between the two compendia. By 1960 legitimate questions began to be asked as to "Why two separate compendia?" and "What is the difference between these two compendia?" Several events then occurred that greatly accelerated and intensified this questioning process.

First, the NF Board approved a dramatic change in its drug admissions policy: no longer would "extent of use" carry any weight as a criterion for acceptance; in its place "therapeutic value" would become the sole determining factor in deciding upon acceptance of non-USP recognized articles for inclusion in the NF.

Second, a major revolution took place in thinking as to drug testing and standardization. In particular, so-called "wet chemical" procedures were replaced with modern instrumental methods involving ultraviolet and infrared spectrophotometry, nuclear magnetic resonance, mass spectrometry, and a host of other sophisticated instrumentation. In turn, these procedures generally required the use of reference standard samples to be run in parallel with the test sample.

Third, an unprecedented change in personnel and philosophy took place in government and particularly at the FDA. Formerly, the FDA leadership had all "come up the ladder" through the ranks of inspectors who knew, understood, and revered the official compendia. New people, brought into the agency in the late 1960s, lacked an appreciation of the value of an outside, independent source of drug standards. In its place, they envisioned the simplicity of government doing all, and the attractiveness of total control that would result from having both drug standardization and enforcement within government's domain.

Fourth, a confluence of factors ranging from public drug reimbursement programs to brand versus generic drug wars led to the establishment of several review groups under governmental auspices for the express purpose of reexamining the total picture of drug standards establishment. Principal among these bodies were the HEW Task Force on Prescription Drugs and the OTA Review Panel on Bioequivalence.

Matching Resources to Needs

The major advances in testing technology and instrumentation that were referred to above contributed to a financial and manpower crunch that was unprecedented in NF-USP history. Moreover, the changing pattern of grant money support and of research interests among faculty members at schools of pharmacy further contributed to the reduced pool of qualified people available as volunteers in compendial work. The obvious result was fewer people and less resources at a time when the demand was rapidly escalating for both. A natural and attractive solution was to combine those resources to make it reasonably possible to meet the immediate and pressing needs.

This solution was further encouraged by a perception on the part of some outside observers that not only was there a degree of duplication of effort with two separate compendia but that there might be some wasted effort due to competition and rivalry between the two compendial operations. This perception was never established in fact, but its very existence did serve as a further spur to thinking along the lines of combining resources.

Compendial Merger: First Considerations

Before any thought or consideration was given to the terms of a possible merger, the concept itself—along with all its advantages and disadvantages—had to be thoroughly explored and weighed. In contrast to the average business operation that is the subject of a sale of purchase, both the NF and USP were unusual—indeed, unique—properties that had professional, scientific, and legal connotations, among others.

American medicine and pharmacy were properly proud of their official compendia, the only such non-governmental drug standards regulating operations in the world. Moreover, the entire United States Pharmacopeial Convention existed solely to produce the USP, while the NF was the profession of pharmacy's very own prime jewel. Many prominent people had contributed extensively during their careers to advance one or the other of these two compendia and to foster its status, recognition, and heritage.

Arguments had long been made by their respective advocates that the scientific competition between the USP and NF was a healthy and beneficial factor that forced both of them to put forth their best efforts. Other advocates of maintaining their separate status argued that the compendia had slightly different philosophies and approaches to solving standards-related problems that would be lost in any amalgamation. Finally, both compendia enjoyed legal rec-

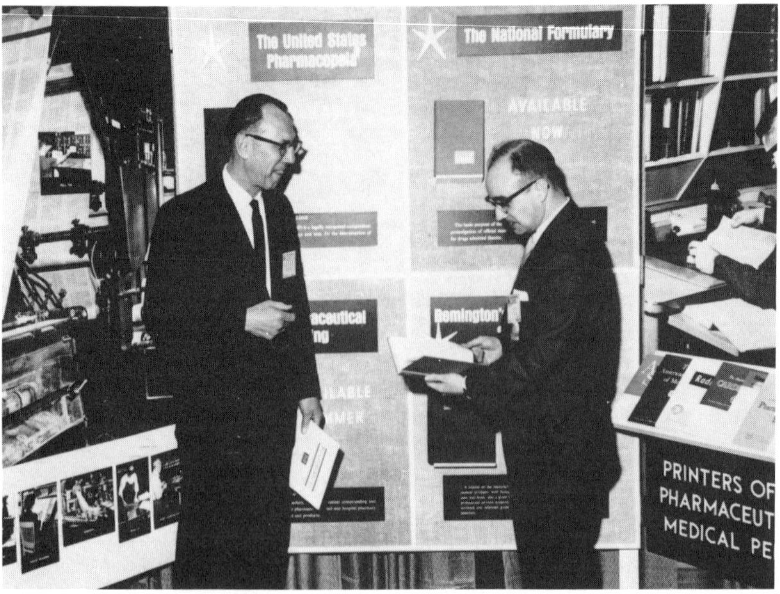

Figure 3. *NF XII—with its dramatic new criteria concerning which drugs would be included—was published in early 1965 and USP XVII was published in mid-1965. The Mack Publishing Company, as official distributor of both compendia, sponsored an exhibit at the 1965 APhA Annual Meeting in Detroit, Michigan. Almost as a forecast of the merger that would take place a decade later, the exhibit co-featured the two new editions. Pictured above, at the exhibit, are USP Director Lloyd C. Miller (l.) and NF Director Edward G. Feldmann (r.).*

ognition under federal and state laws. Would this status be jeopardized, or even lost, if their basic status were tinkered with in any material way?

Hence, the earliest discussions of possible compendial merger were devoted almost exclusively to these ancillary, but yet fundamental, side issues. This contrasted markedly with a typical business acquisition or merger in which financial issues are the initial point of discussion. It also helps to explain why the subject of NF-USP merger—and the discussions on that subject—appeared to consume an inordinate amount of time before that objective was eventually achieved.

Merger Negotiations: Chronological Highlights

Interestingly, the first serious suggestion of a NF-USP merger (of which this speaker is aware) came from a prominent physician member of the USP Board of Trustees. Windsor Cutting, in a USP "Pre-

Convention Conference" on March 28, 1960, presented a paper titled "The Pharmacopeia and the Physician," in which he had a sub-section headed "Multiplicity of Publications." He devoted several paragraphs to the subject, but his general theme can be summed up by quoting two key sentences from his paper: "It well may be asked whether amalgamation of the USP with the NF would not simplify use and allow economy of format. . . . Although ownership and traditions are different, I believe that it would be worthwhile to discuss the possibility with representatives of the NF."

The suggestion from Dr. Cutting appeared to lie dormant for the next few years, although apparently it was at least informally discussed within USP circles. Indeed, the first real mention of compendial merger to appear in the pharmacy press was a story in the April 5, 1965, issue of *Drug News Weekly.* Accompanying a photo of USP's Lloyd C. Miller and NF's Edward G. Feldmann—each with the just published USP XVII and NF XII—was a brief article headlined "Eventual Merger with NF Likely, USP Official Says." Dr. Miller is then quoted in the article as saying that "some very serious people have made the suggestion" of NF-USP merger, and that "you will see some interesting things happening in the next three years or so." And, in fact, Dr. Miller's prediction proved to be accurate. Specifically, Drs. Miller and Feldmann discussed the matter sufficiently in private to convince Feldmann that Miller and USP were serious in at least exploring the possibility of compendial merger. On this basis, Feldmann proposed that the governing boards of both responsible organizations appoint official representatives to initiate formal discussions.

In a letter dated January 12, 1967, Dr. Miller wrote to the head of the APhA, William S. Apple, to follow up on this initiative. In part Miller's letter stated: "Last November, Dr. Feldmann informed me that he was asking the APhA [Board of Trustees] to consider naming a committee to look into [the topic of merger] and suggested that a similar action by the USP might be in order. I agreed and the USP Board of Trustees has set up a committee . . . of Dr. Tice, Dr. Klumpp, and myself." The APhA Board acted concurrently on Dr. Feldmann's recommendation, and named Hugo Schaefer, Apple, and Feldmann as a three-person team to represent APhA's interests.

Meetings began shortly thereafter accompanied by a blaze of publicity in the pharmacy press. As one typical example, the July 31, 1967, issue of *American Druggist* carried its lead article under the banner "USP and NF Leaders Confer on 'Consolidation' Measures." The six representatives continued to meet periodically over the next year or so, but progress was painfully slow as the big issues involved continued to be insurmountable stumbling blocks.

Then the negotiations—which had remained highly cordial throughout—gradually came to a stand-still as efforts were concentrated on producing the 1970 editions of the two compendia. In addition, Dr. Miller had announced his decision to take early retirement, and USP attention was further diverted to selecting his successor and to the related transition in USP directorship. The USP Convention of 1970 subsequently refocused attention on the merger proposition via comments in several officers' reports and resolutions passed by the assembled delegates. Indeed, the newly installed USP President and Board Chairman were quoted in the press as believing "they had a mandate from the USP Convention" to achieve a merger.

In a departure from the joint six-person committee that had functioned before, the two boards assigned the USP and NF staffs the task of working out a proposal for a "joint venture." Hence, not only was the operational format changed, but a new unification concept was advanced, namely, a "joint venture." In retrospect, this introduced a highly complex solution to achieve what procedurally should have been a simple "merger." However, the "joint venture" concept was visualized as enabling both groups to remain in existence, to keep their respective identities and traditions, but to produce a single end-product. Although this joint venture approach had considerable political appeal, in practice it could not be translated into a workable formula despite long and dedicated efforts by the respective staff people.

How close this did come, however, can be seen from a letter from Heller to Apple dated July 10, 1972, in which Heller reported three actions by the USP Board the first of which was: "The (USP) Board formally reviewed and voted disapproval of creation of a new organization to operate the USP and NF as you and Dr. Feldmann and Dr. Moyer and I had spelled it out in meetings this Spring." This rejection was a sudden and unexpected disappointment; indeed it constituted a set-back of major proportions.

Lack of tangible progress quickly led to deep frustration for all concerned and signs of acrimony began to surface for the first time during the entire history of merger negotiations. The high point of this frustration level came when the USP delegates petitioned for a special meeting of the USP Convention which was subsequently convened on April 14, 1973. The special meeting proved to be emotional but also inconclusive—at least concerning any action on the merger issue. However, it did serve to get the discussions "back on track."

But, again, the negotiations started to bog down when neither side was willing to accord a controlling interest to the other and at the same time realized that a "co-equals" structure probable would not work either because no one would really be in control. Suddenly, however, the impasse was broken on March 26, 1974, when APhA President George D. Denmark sent a "fish or cut bait" letter to USP in which for the first time was suggested the possibility of a simple, straightforward purchase arrangement.

The USP Board immediately reacted positively to this outright purchase approach and less than four months later full agreement was reached and announced to the outside world. Press releases dated July 5, 1974, from both APhA and USPC, proclaimed the good news.

The formal ceremonies to complete the transaction took place on the following first business day of the new year, January 2, 1975. This was virtually the same date that the very first steps toward USP I had been taken 155 years earlier, back on January 1, 1820—a truly fitting climax to a most historic occasion. If it could ever be accurately said that "an idea whose time had come" was fulfilled, this phrase describes the dramatic event of NF-USP merger.

Conclusion

In the course of my review I have touched upon most of the various *controversies*—or at least the primary ones—that arose and had to be resolved during the merger negotiations. It is now much more simple to address the *consequences.*

The merged USP-NF not only has survived in the face of outside attacks during the ensuing decade, but it has thrived. It is stronger and more viable then ever before. Dr. Heller and his staff—some from the old USP staff, some from the old NF and Drug Standards Laboratory staff, and some entirely new people—have done a superb job of advancing the standards and status of the merged compendia.

More than ever before, the USP-NF today is the acknowledged world-wide leader in drug standards and specifications. Over the years the high quality of drugs in the American marketplace has been due in large measure to the USP and NF standing behind them. In 1988 that situation is more a reality than ever before.

The Recent History and the Future of the NF Concept

by William M. Heller

What the NF purchase boiled down to at the very end of the negotiations was a pair of the most basic factors: survival and money. Let's listen to a tape of the meeting of the USP Board of Trustees via a telephone conference call on July 3, 1974 in which they agreed to buy the NF and the equipment of the Drug Standards Laboratory.

The players were physicians Paul L. McLain, chairman; John H. Moyer, president; George E. Farrar, vice-president; and Walter Modell; pharmacists Paul F. Parker, treasurer, Leslie L. Eisenbrandt, William J. Kinnard, Fred T. Mahaffey, and Linwood F. Tice; and attorney Joseph Valentino. The meeting was about 45 minutes long, so I shall be giving you only a few minutes of selected portions. First, there was lengthy discussion of the terms of the proposed agreement worked out between Dr. Apple and me, then a new factor—survival itself—was sprung on them.

FRED MAHAFFEY: Could I bring up a point which is . . .

PAUL MCLAIN: Who is speaking?

MAHAFFEY: Mahaffey. I talked to someone this morning and then confirmed this with Joe Valentino. I have heard rumors that were substantiated with my conversation with this gentleman this morning. He has talked to Jim Doluisio, the Dean at the Texas College of Pharmacy, who is a member of the Committee on Bioavailability of [Senator Edward] Kennedy. He has indicated that the Committee's recommendation to Senator Kennedy was that the USP and NF be abandoned or abolished or something to this effect and that this responsibility then be placed in the hands of the FDA. I would like Bill to comment on what he has heard.

LINWOOD TICE: Fred, are you talking about bioavailability or setting all standards?

WILLIAM HELLER: Everything. The information I have is that the report will suggest that—well, it will state outright that the volunteer system of USP and NF as it now exists is passe; that to do what they envision needs doing would take a major overhaul and upgrading of the USP and NF system; and although they admit that that is possible, they don't raise any hope for it. Then they speculate about a new organization which would be—could be—non-governmental but would be government-funded; and just how it would tie into the FDA, whether it would be a part of FDA, whether it would be a part of HEW, or outside of both and actually even non-governmental. So they don't preclude the kind of organization that USP and NF together are, but they do say that the work that needs doing would take funding beyond what is available to the USP and NF now.

TICE: I think the problem there is that there has been friction between the Academy of Pharmaceutical Sciences and the APhA official family concerning the importance of bioavailability. That has been very awkward; but if we acquire the National Formulary, the APhA will have no further vested interest in bioavailability testing and I think this is going to eliminate the problem. I think Jim Doluisio is embarrassed because the Academy has not been able to see eye to eye with APhA as an official group. That's just a complex, technical question. But I think it all has to do with bioavailability. It has nothing to do with all of the standards of the USP and NF by any means.

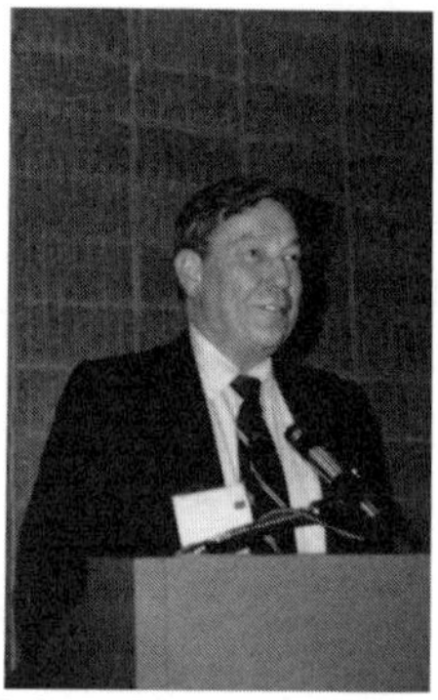

William M. Heller, Ph.D., *has been Executive Director of the USP since 1970 and is, constitutionally, chairman of the USP Committee of Revision. He has served on the faculties of pharmacy and medicine at the University of Arkansas and is currently Adjunct Professor of Pharmacy at the University of Maryland. He was director of the Department of Scientific Services of the American Society of Hospital Pharmacists and editor of the American Hospital Formulary Service before joining the USP staff in 1968. Dr. Heller has been the recipient of many awards and honors, including the Harvey A.K. Whitney Award of the ASHP, the Rho Chi Lecture Award, and the Remington Honor Medal.*

HELLER: Linwood, I don't want to say *how* I know, but I know it *does*.

TICE: It does?

HELLER: Yes, it talks about the whole kit and kaboodle.

TICE: Do you really think FDA is prepared to take over the USP and the NF?

HELLER: No.

TICE: I don't think they want any part of it.

HELLER: But I think this report will say that—that this is something that needs to be done.

MAHAFFEY: Once you announce the fact that the USP has purchased the NF and that the Drug Standards Laboratory and all these functions will now be under one organization—won't this be a good case to take to the government in terms of—or to take to Kennedy—as a result of this report?

HELLER: My answer would be that, yes, we are the organization they are talking about. We are building ourselves to be in a position to do what they want done and then it will be up to this Board to decide how much involvement with government funding you might want to have.

TICE: That's the only hope of getting it. We will never get it as long as there is a schism between the two groups.

HELLER: That is exactly my feeling.

* * *

There was then a long, long discussion of the need to persuade Dr. Apple that USP ought to be able to escape from the contract for the purchase of the NF if the government decided to take over the NF. I reported that such an escape clause was in one of our proposals and that Dr. Apple's attitude was that:

HELLER: He wasn't going to guarantee anything. We know what we're getting. It's a judgment on our part that it's worth it or not. I think that's just about the words he used: it's a business judgment on our part.

TICE: We're willing to go through with our bargain, but if all we're buying is an empty shell, I don't see how he can expect us to go on paying for it for ten years.

McLain: Well, we all lose. He loses, too, even if he does nothing.

William Kinnard: Bill Heller, are you going to have a joint press release on this?

Tice: Bill, Heller, this is Tice again. Don't you think we are proper in talking to Bill about this eventuality? I can't believe he would take the illogical position where you buy a pig in a poke, where you buy it whether it turns out good or not. If it doesn't turn out well, he would lose the NF anyhow. It isn't like he'd be giving away some assets that he would have otherwise.

Heller: I think the whole subject ought to be discussed in a Board meeting of ours. What it boils down to is, What do we do as an organization if we don't have the Pharmacopeia? Do we even want to exist? And if so, for what? Because that's what we're talking about here.

Walter Modell: No, we're talking about buying something.

Heller: Well, our reservation is "the government declaring its intention to take over the NF." If we own the NF, our reimbursement from the government is not going to be any less for owning the NF. It would be more.

Tice: Do you think the government would reimburse us for loss of assets if they took over?

Heller: I don't know if they would. But regardless, we only have one purpose for existence and that's to do the USP—and the NF—so, I just can't understand how we could talk about this at the lawyer level without having the Board meet and discuss it fully ahead of time so that we would have some idea of what the attorneys should be trying to do.

Tice: Well, Bill, I think they are related, but I don't think they are the same thing. We're buying the NF, that's one thing. If we're talking about what's going to happen if USP folds, that's something else. They may be related. It would seem to me that if we began the procedure of buying the National Formulary, and then the National Formulary was taken out of existence, then further payments for something that no longer existed would be unreasonable.

Heller: I'm assuming that at that point the USP Convention would also go out of existence. But that's something the Board has to figure out.

Tice: But would the individual members of the Board be held responsible for a professional obligation made when we were in business?

JOE VALENTINO: Usually—this is Joe Valentino—just off the top of my head, usually a Board of Trustees member is not liable for poor business judgment. Usually, there has to be something in addition to the poor business judgment. The courts aren't going to concern themselves with poor business judgment. There has to be some aspect of fraud involved, or bad faith, or something like that, and that's when they would hold a Director liable. Without that, they usually don't look into the question of poor business judgment. The question of bankruptcy, in either event would probably—well, first of all, the way I see it, if you don't buy the NF, USPC is doomed and if you do buy the NF you've got a fighting chance. If the government should come in and take over the assets of the USP and NF—which is highly unlikely—they would compensate you. More likely, they'd just wipe you out of the Food Drug and Cosmetic Act, which would be, in a sense, like changing the zoning law and would not be taking of property and they would not have to compensate you. In which case you would be bankrupt and at that time, probably, because of our incorporation under the old D.C. statutes, they would probably distribute [the assets] under the bankruptcy laws; and then the remainder funds, if any, would probably go to similar organizations. The court would decide what a "similar organization" would be.

TICE: Joe Valentino, do you think we're off-base in trying to put forward an escape clause with APhA?

Here the tape ended and we start the next one in mid-sentence.

VALENTINO: . . . on its merits. Without it, you lose.

TICE: If we went bankrupt he wouldn't get his money anyhow.

VALENTINO: Well, it would no doubt be secured but he would stand in line with the rest of the creditors and probably he would make out as well as possible. So to my way of thinking, it's just a question of losing 100% or having a fighting chance in which you may win or lose. What's the difference if you lose? If you're going to go bankrupt, you might as well go down bankrupt swinging—that's my opinion. I'm sorry to inject my personal opinion and not to stick to legal opinion.

TICE: Oh, I agree we're in a stronger position with it than we are without it.

LESLIE EISENBRANDT: It seems that by what Joe has just said then, that although it would be wise to look into this, the probability is that we can go ahead regardless. It looks as if—if we don't, we're going to lose any other way, any direction we may go.

MAHAFFEY: Mr. Chairman.

McLAIN: Yes, Fred.

MAHAFFEY: Why don't you outline a consensus for us so we can make our votes known here.

McLAIN: Are you ready to talk in these terms, gentlemen?

______: Yes, Sir. Yes. Yes.

McLAIN: My proposal for consensus is that we agree, subject to mail or telegram confirmation official vote, on the terms which have been outlined for the purchase of the NF by Dr. Heller; that in addition such exploration of the possibility of an escape clause as may seem at all feasible or likely to be profitable be pursued. But that our agreement not be contingent upon that. Is this the position you're willing to support now after having heard about it?

TICE: Very well stated.

MAHAFFEY: I would approve—Mahaffey.

McLAIN: Mahaffey, all right.

MODELL: Are you calling the roll?

McLAIN: Yes. Let's call the roll.

HELLER: Oh, I don't have the roll here.

McLAIN: Well, just speak up. We'll mark them down.

MODELL: Modell approves.

McLAIN: Modell approves.

FARRAR: Farrar approves.

McLAIN: Farrar approves.

KINNARD: Kinnard approves.

McLAIN: Kinnard approves.

EISENBRANDT: Eisenbrandt approves.

McLAIN: Eisenbrandt approves.

TICE: Tice approves.

McLAIN: Tice approves.

MAHAFFEY: Mahaffey approves.

McLAIN: Mahaffey up.

PARKER: Parker approves.

McLAIN: Parker approves.

HELLER: Moyer approve?

MOYER: Yes.

McLAIN: McLain approves.

HELLER: McLain approves. That is all, Mr. Chairman. Dr. DeGraff is not here.

McLAIN: Oh, DeGraff is not on. Is there any other business we need to take up?

EISENBRANDT: But Bill will also check with people in FDA to see if we can get a reading [on their views]. And Bill Heller, are you going to make inquiry to Apple about the escape clause—even though nothing may come of it?

HELLER: I will bring to his attention that the Board wishes us to pursue that in any way we can, as we get this thing into legal language.

MAHAFFEY: This is Mahaffey. What about the news release now?

TICE: I would be against that. I'd be against a news release that's one-sided. I think we should hold back on a news release if we can possibly do it at this point.

MODELL: I think it ought to be a joint release.

TICE: I think maybe in a week or so, but I think this is a little premature to put out a news release.

McLAIN: I don't think we should put out a news release until both boards have officially approved and it can be worked out. Certainly it should be joint.

HELLER: I don't think that Dr. Apple cares to issue joint releases but we will work one out that would have the same wording issued from both places.

McLAIN: OK, that will be satisfactory.

HELLER: Now the reason we've been in this hurry is to have this information known at the time of Senator Kennedy's press conference next Wednesday or Thursday, so that when people read about that new proposed compendial organization there, they'll know that something is happening at USP and NF to get in line. So I would hate to have to issue a release *after* that press conference—which sounds like we have scrambled to change things around to get there. We would like to at least appear to be in step.

TICE: I think it would take a lot of wind out of the Kennedy sails on the Compendium if we could do it.

HELLER: So if Dr. Apple and I could get together on Friday, I would like to go ahead and issue the news release.

MCLAIN: Since there is some timing problem on that, I would withdraw my objection to waiting for the official mail vote.

TICE: So will I.

KINNARD: OK.

EISENBRANDT: Paul McLain, I wanted to—you've been very cautious in your reactions to all of this. Are you—are you wholeheartedly behind this?

MCLAIN: Yes, I am now.

EISENBRANDT: OK.

EISENBRANDT: It seems to me that we have sort of delayed and maneuvered for a period of four years or less without coming to a head. Anytime there is a head, there is always a hard decision to make. It seems to me that we are probably making a very good choice. In my own mind I don't know all the finances of it and I am trusting the rest of you who have been exploring this in detail. But if we can't make it financially, it all folds up. It's a gamble I suppose, but we might as well take that gamble.

MCLAIN: Well, this whole five years has been a gamble and we have done pretty well.

EISENBRANDT: I feel pretty good about it.

MCLAIN: Any other comments? Shall we adjourn, then?
Yes. Good bye.

Unfortunately, John Moyer's telephone connection was so poor that one could hardly hear him, so he gave up trying to speak. John had been the Board's chief negotiator with APhA and I'm sure he would have had much to say.

But wasn't that a remarkable meeting? Not one raised voice. Not one harsh or bitter word. Just mature discussion, even though the negotiations with APhA had been less than harmonious over the years and now fate had thrown in the fatal threat from Congress' Office of Technology Assessment report.

Two days later, on July 5, USP issued two news releases. When Senator Kennedy's Committee held its press conference on the OTA report the following week, we distributed our news releases to the attendees. Two of the nongovernmental experts who served on the OTA Committee later became members of the USPC Board of Trustees: Fred Shideman was elected vice president the next year, president in 1980, and served as past president from 1985 until his death in 1988. Jim Doluiso was elected to the Board for the 1985–1990 term.

In our news releases we were not contesting the OTA report. We were declaring that we were right in step with it. One news release announced the purchase of the NF.[1] The second called upon the professions, government, and industry to "take advantage of this unique opportunity to help create a strong and modern compendial organization to serve the needs of the public," stating that it would be a mistake to assume that unification of the compendia was an end in itself. "It is crucial to meet the emerging new challenges involving the nation's drug supply with a parallel new organizational approach having the versatility, breadth, and knowledge to do the job," I was quoted as saying.

What the report actually recommended was this:[2]

> A single organization capable of setting standards adequate to assure the quality and uniform bioavailability of drug products should be established to replace the present USP and NF as the official standard-setting organization of the federal government.

In the explanation of this recommendation, they said:

> Several options are readily apparent for the location of the new organization: within the FDA but separate from the compliance-monitoring group, within HEW but separate from FDA, or outside of the Federal Government as an independent organization. The possibility that the USP and the NF could merge and make sufficient changes in their structures and functions to fulfill the criteria for an effective standard-setting organization is not precluded, but the changes necessary would be extensive.

No government agency ever talked to us openly and specifically in following up on the OTA report. Certainly, FDA must have held internal discussions, but they did not include us in those discussions. Commissioner Schmidt and Bureau of Drugs Director Crout posed with APhA and USPC officials at the formal signing of the contract to purchase the NF.[3] Within the Bureau of Drugs, both a policy group and an operations group were formed to provide a continuing liaison with USP-NF, adding agency commitment to the revision process in addition to the person-to-person relationship that had long been our working arrangement. So we know from their actions that FDA has been generally supportive, and that is what counts.

Of course, in all this nondiscussion with government agencies, the possibility of government funds for USPC went undiscussed, too. From our standpoint, we never pursued it. We have believed that standards-setting should be carried out without government grants and/or industry subsidy if possible, so that there would be no undue influence on that score.

And we have not gone bankrupt. True, Dr. Apple had figured out every cent we had and could expect to make for the next ten years, and asked for it. And I had it figured out, too, thought it was worth it, and so I said OK. But the unspoken part of those calculations and negotiations was the ability to raise prices. The reference standards programs of both USP and NF had been operated as necessary nuisances, nowhere near recovering their share of the costs of operating the revision programs. Once both programs were consolidated, we had the critical mass to improve exponentially on the reference standards operation—and price it accordingly. Since then, half of our revenues have come from reference standards and half from books.

What about the books? The Food, Drug and Cosmetic Act does not mirror the self-imposed division of responsibility into USP "best drugs" and NF "second best drugs." The tests and standards in each book are equally enforceable by the FDA. We could include all monographs in only one of the books and eliminate the other title or save it for something else, as far as the FD&C Act is concerned.

The reasons for actively using the NF title are mostly legal. It was feared that the NF name could be used by someone else, if we did not continue to use it ourselves. Since the name appears in so many state laws as well as national laws, it seemed unreasonable to expect that we could get all of those laws changed. So the conclusion was that we should keep both titles alive.

On the other hand, one of the problems that led to the merger negotiations in the first place was the switching of drugs back and forth between the books from one revision period to another. A borderline drug might have to be relabeled as either USP or NF every five years, a nuisance and a cost to the manufacturers.

Thus, the basic question to be faced concerned the utility of the USP Scope program: the selection of those drugs "most fully established and best understood," to quote the Preface of the 1820 Pharmacopeia. After 155 years, what was its influence in encouraging practitioners to select USP drugs as the best drugs?

The 1962 Kefauver-Harris Amendments to the FD&C Act had given the FDA the authority to prevent drugs from being marketed until their efficacy, as well as safety, was proven. Furthermore, the Amendments directed the FDA to go all the way back to the passage of the Act in 1938 to review the drugs that had been marketed under the New Drug requirements for safety, alone. If the FDA was going to rule off the market those drugs that were not efficacious, the need for the USP to make a judgment in order to influence professional opinions may have been diminished.

At the meeting of the Pharmacopeial Convention right after the purchase of the NF, in 1975, the Convention adopted a resolution to the effect that the Committee of Revision should set standards for all drugs. "All" drugs—not just the best drugs.[4]

Ken Barker, who had been on the USP staff in the early 1970s and laid the groundwork for the USP-NF negotiations with a "white paper," wrote another one, on the USP Scope program. The recommendation was that the narrow Scope program should be eliminated. Rather, the Committee of Revision could consider providing a medical use commentary on all drugs, as well as set standards for them. The Board of Trustees and the Committee of Revision accepted these challenges and the following decisions were made:

- The USP and NF would be published in one physical book, if possible.
- USP would contain all drug products and drug substances.
- NF would contain pharmaceutic ingredients — inactive ingredients, excipients. Thus, it would be unlikely that a drug would pass from USP to NF or vice versa, in the future.
- The "dispensing information" that had been included in the 1975 USP in abbreviated form in the monographs of drugs used in ambulatory care would be expanded in content and to cover all drugs. Subsequently, the Board decided to publish it outside the USP itself and called it USP Dispensing Information, later shortened to USP DI.

These decisions drastically changed the nature of the USPC organization in almost every facet.

In accepting the goal of setting standards for all drugs, the Committee of Revision has in ten years added as many monographs as were in USP or NF at the time of the merger. The priorities for expansion have been:[5]

(1) Every new drug marketed in 1975 and thereafter would be included.

(2) All articles included in USP XIX and NF XIV and their Supplements would be included as long as they remained on the market.

(3) Other drugs marketed before 1975 and deemed by the Subcommittee on Scope to be among the more medically useful would be included.

(4) All marketed dosage forms of any drug substance already admitted would be included.

(5) Combinations among the 300 most frequently prescribed drugs in the U.S.A. would be included, along with any components thereof not already included.

(6) The most important and frequently used pharmaceutic ingredients, as determined by the Subcommittee on Formulations, would be included.

About a thousand unfinished monographs are in the system at any point in time. Thus the total workload is four times what it was for USP alone.

This is a major change in the workload of both the USP Committee of Revision and the staff. The 60-member Committee of Revision has been expanded steadily and now numbers 95. The number of Advisory Panels has tripled, to 34.

Committee members no longer have the time to go into their laboratories and test something out for themselves. They have become decision-makers, making their decisions in response to data supplied to them by others.

In addition to the greatly increased paper-handling chores, staff has had to gear up a laboratory operation to support the reference standards program and to serve as an independent source of data for the Committee. We have increased from about 40 staff people at the time of consolidation to about 140; we have grown beyond the point where any one person can be up to date on all the revision proposals and discussions.

As I mentioned, we did not actively seek government funds for our USP-NF and USP DI operations. We did, however, include government agencies among those with whom we touched base—"touched" is the appropriate word for fund raising—touched as sources of funds in a one-time, non-recurring expansion of the Laboratory. Pharmacist S. Blake Yates, who had had a most successful retirement job as fund-raiser for the Auburn University School of Pharmacy, assumed the task of raising a million dollars for the expansion and equipment of the new Drug Research and Testing Laboratory and for getting the new manpower on stream. We postulated that a four-year program would do it and that the organization would then be able to carry on at a new level. Mr. Yates did raise the million dollars, thanks in large measure to AMA's $300,000. Almost all the rest came from the pharmaceutical industry. None came from government. And none came from major pharmacy organizations. As expected, the four years proved sufficient for us to rearrange our financial structure so that we could continue to operate the Laboratory at its new level, which has grown to about twenty full-time chemists.

One of the hassles in the merger negotiations was over the inclusion in USP and NF of information other than tests and standards of strength, quality, and purity. Doses had been introduced into USP in 1900. Categories of use, strengths commercially available, and various kinds of notes to the maker and to the dispenser had been introduced over the years, culminating in the dispensing information section of the monographs in the 1975 USP. With the separate publication of USP DI, however, USP and NF have become "clean". There is no longer an effort to make them more useful to the pharmacist by including non-standards information.

As a matter of fact, that long contest for the pharmacists' attention has gone the other way: in the 1988 USP DI dosage form monographs, there is a paragraph summarizing the USP requirements for that dosage form!

Financially, USP DI and USP-NF have been priced so that a state that decides to switch its purchase requirements will be just as supportive of USPC by requiring USP DI as by requiring USP-NF to be present in a pharmacy.

Although the removal of doses, categories of use, and other non-standards-setting information from USP-NF was generally desired, there was considerable apprehension over the expansion of that type of information in the forthcoming USP DI. There was no secret about what the Committee of Revision planned to do. Draft monographs were published and widely distributed for comment.

At one time or another in the three years of preparation of the first edition of USP DI, every major organization in the pharmacopeial arena had an objection. APhA was the loudest, protesting that dispensing information in the USP would be looked at as so official that state boards would enforce it. ASHP said the same thing more quietly. NARD said state boards of pharmacy should cease requiring the book. AMA worked behind the scenes. It objected to the basic thrust of USP DI, that the pharmacist should advise the patient about prescription drugs. AMA said the pharmacist should not be injected into the patient/physician interface. FDA and PMA were concerned that dispensing information in the USP itself might be misinterpreted as coming under USP's labeling authority in the FD&C Act, even though the information was in a separate part of the monograph.

Some of these concerns were solved by the decision to publish dispensing information in a separate book and not entitle it as a part of the official Pharmacopeia. The AMA decided it was preferable to have the biprofessional USP advising the pharmacist what to tell the patient than to have a pharmacy organization doing it alone later, if the counseling movement strengthened.

The USP DI history epitomizes the pricelessness of an independent compendial organization where physicians and pharmacists and health care practitioners and scientists of all kinds can get together on behalf of the public, rather than as representatives of professions or organizations seeking to protect and promote themselves.

In sum, the NF purchase by USPC was a win-win event for all concerned. APhA collected over $2,000,000 from the sale of NF and the Drug Standards Laboratory equipment, plus the revenues from the sale of NF XIV. USPC, in addition to being recognized as the sole standards-setting agency for drugs, was freed from keeping in lock-step with another organization as it pursued additional activities where medicine, pharmacy, government, and industry work together for the public welfare.

A postscript: what happened to the people? In mergers some people usually lose their jobs. Not in this case. All three full-time NF employees and all of the Laboratory employees were offered the opportunity to join the USP staff. NF Director John Bergen decided instead to take the presidency of the Philadelphia College of Pharmacy and Science; he took Christine Bailey with him. Charles Barnstein did join the USP staff and is now Assistant Director, Drug Standards Revision, Drug Standards Division. He serves under Lee T. Grady, who has been promoted from director of the laboratory to director of the Drug Standards Division and is in charge of the whole USP and NF revision program from the staff standpoint. Bob King was a chemist in the Drug Standards Laboratory and is now Assistant Director, Technical Services, Drug Standards Division. One other DSL chemist, Vivian Gray, is still with the laboratory after 18 years. Truly, these people have contributed much to making this merger a win-win situation for all of us.

Finally, for the NF buffs, be it known that in the USPC business office, USP-NF is referred to solely as the NF. With USAN and the USP Dictionary of Drug Names and USP DI to keep track of as well, they have dropped the "USP" part of all titles and refer to each by its added appellation; thus, USAN, DI—and NF.

References

1. "The 1970's—changing directions," *Abstract of Proceedings of the U.S. Pharmacopeial Convention, Inc., Washington, DC. April 14, 1973; March 22, 1975; April 17–19, 1980.* (Rockville, MD: Board of Trustees, U.S. Pharmacopeial Convention, Inc., 1981), pp. 72–74.
2. Ibid., p. 194.
3. Ibid., p. 6.
4. Ibid., p. 229.
5. Ibid., p. 389.

Selected Pages
from

THE

NATIONAL FORMULARY

OF

UNOFFICINAL PREPARATIONS.

FIRST ISSUE.

BY AUTHORITY OF THE
AMERICAN PHARMACEUTICAL ASSOCIATION.

PUBLISHED BY THE AMERICAN PHARMACEUTICAL ASSOCIATION.
1888.

THE

NATIONAL FORMULARY

OF

UNOFFICINAL PREPARATIONS.

FIRST ISSUE.

BY AUTHORITY OF THE

AMERICAN PHARMACEUTICAL ASSOCIATION.

PUBLISHED BY THE AMERICAN PHARMACEUTICAL ASSOCIATION.
1888.

PREFACE.

It is well known that the remedies for which the Pharmacopœia prescribes definite standards, constitute only a limited portion of the resources of the medical profession in the treatment of the sick. Without referring to the more ephemeral preparations, or to such as are of a proprietary character, or are used by the public for self-medication, there is a large number of others, which are more or less frequently prescribed by physicians, or demanded by the public, but which are not recognized by the Pharmacopœia, either because they were not deemed by the revisers to be of sufficient importance to be included in the official work, or because they originated subsequently to the appearance of that work, or for other reasons. Owing to the absence of an authoritative standard, many of these unofficial preparations have been, and are being made, after different formulæ, and in varying strength, so that the pharmacists, particularly in the larger cities, are compelled to procure and keep on hand a variety of brands of what is intended to be one and the same preparation, to satisfy the demands of their patrons, professional or otherwise. The evils arising from this condition of things are so well known and so far-reaching in their results, that there is no need of any argument in favor of a plan which may palliate the existing evil, chiefly caused by a lack of uniformity, or the want of a common standard.

In order to bring about a practical amelioration of this state of things, a local Committee representing the College of Pharmacy of the City of New York, the Kings County Pharmaceutical Society of Brooklyn, and the German Apothecaries' Society of the City of New York, several years ago published a book of formulæ, comprising those which were in most frequent use in their immediate vicinity, and recommended the same to the medical profession. As this book appeared at a time which happened to be particularly favorable to the realization of the object sought to be attained, it gained so much ground, even outside of the locality for which it was originally intended, that the Joint Committee, authorized by the Societies which it represented, tendered the work to the American Pharmaceutical Association, at the Annual Meeting held at Pittsburgh, in 1885, as a nucleus for the construction of a National Formulary. The Association having accepted the gift, a Committee was appointed to prepare such a work, and as a first result, this Committee presented at the next Annual Meeting, held at Providence, in 1886, a "*Preliminary Draft of a National Formulary*," comprising whatever the Committee had been able to gather, either from existing formularies, or from its own labors, or from the special contributions of individuals or societies. This Draft showed, more forcibly than could have been done in any other manner, how serious the existing evil was, and at the same time, how difficult would be the task to bring into harmony the conflicting views and customs. For the purpose of enabling the Committee to accomplish this task with better expectation of success, it was enlarged by the addition of one member from every State Pharmaceutical Association in the United States and Canada.

The Committee thus constituted has endeavored, to the best of its ability, to carry out the object for which it was appointed. While it was, of course, impossible for most of the members representing other States, personally to attend the weekly meetings of the Committee, held in New York City, yet all important matters were referred to them by circular, and their votes thereon solicited, so that the results, regarded as a whole, truly represent the intentions and decisions of the whole Committee, though individual members may not have agreed upon every detail.

One of the most difficult problems which the Committee encountered, was the selection of the preparations which should be admitted into the Formulary. In order to ascertain the wishes of the different sections of the country, a printed list of the proposed titles was sent to each member, and a vote or expression of opinion thereon asked for. After all the votes had been returned, it was evident that much would still be left to the discretion of the Editing Sub-Committee, which had in the meantime been appointed. The latter, thereupon, prepared a final list of titles, which was again submitted to the members, and this list having been slightly amended in accordance with the suggestions received, was made the basis of the final text, though in the course of editing some further changes, chiefly additions, became necessary in order to fill in existing gaps. On looking over the contents of the book, every individual reader will probably encounter quite a number of preparations with which he is unfamiliar, or which he has never had occasion to use or to dispense, and the presence of which, from his standpoint, may appear superfluous. It should, however, be remembered that every section of this large country had to be considered; hence, what may be entirely unused or only rarely used in one section, may be of common occurrence in another. It is quite probable that some preparations which ought to have been received into the Formulary have been overlooked, or that some of those introduced are not as frequently employed as has been represented to the Committee. Whatever error may have been committed in one direction or another, will no doubt be corrected in subsequent editions.

While it was at no time contemplated by the Committee as a whole—though, perhaps, by some individual members—to devise imitations of any of the popular nostrums of the present day, yet it was very difficult to decide exactly where the line should be drawn. Consequently the list will be found to include a small number of formulæ which may recall some of the before-mentioned preparations, but which are constructed on rational principles, irrespective of mere external appearance and taste, and mainly with regard to uniform composition and reliable effect. It is not expected that these preparations will readily replace, in the eyes of the public, the much-advertised nostrums, but it is hoped that if proper therapeutic effects are expected from them, they will be used or directed to be used in place of the commercial articles, the composition of which is generally kept secret. A proposition was at one time made to include in the work definitions and descriptions of the more important crude drugs and chemicals which have come into use since the last U. S. Pharmacopœia was issued. But it was found that the labor involved in the task already outlined was so great, that no time could be devoted to any further additions. Hence the project had to be abandoned, though it will be a comparatively easy matter to incorporate these additions in a subsequent edition.

In constructing the formulæ of the compound preparations, it has been the endeavor of the Committee to make them as independent from each other as possible, so that only a comparatively small number of what may be called *basic preparations* need be kept in stock. The principal bases thus required are:

No. 25. Elixir Adjuvans. As a vehicle, chiefly for saline preparations.—No. 31. Aromatic Elixir. Intended to be used as a substitute for the officinal Elixir Aurantii, unless the latter or some other flavored Elixir should be preferred.—No. 42. Elixir of Cinchona.—No. 44. Detannated Elixir of Cinchona.—No. 54. Elixir of Yerba Santa.—No. 81. Elixir of Pepsin.—No. 105. Compound Elixir of Taraxacum.—No. 337. Aromatic Spirit.—No. 338. Compound Spirit of Orange.—No. 340. Spirit of Curaçao.—No. 352. Syrup of Coffee.—No. 360. Aromatic Syrup of Yerba Santa.—No. 394. Detannated Tincture of Cinchona.—If these are kept in stock in reasonable quantities, most of the compound preparations contained in the Formulary may be prepared in a short time.

Regarding the system of weights and measures used in the work, the probable action of the Committee had been foreshadowed in their last Report to the American Pharmaceutical Association, in which they expressed their conviction that all medicines that are prescribed by *measure*, had better be prepared by measure, or by weight *and* measure. The Committee is of the opinion that the working formulæ, either in a Pharmacopœia or in a Formulary, need not all be forced into one rigid, immutable, and uniform system of weights or of measures, but that a judicious and common-sense selection of one or another system, in different formulæ of the same work, may be perfectly legitimate, so long as those used in one and the same formula are practically commensurate with each other—the object, in all cases, being to obtain uniform and definite products, the relative strength of which will be immediately understood without special calculations. While, therefore, the system of *parts by weight* has been unreservedly admitted in the case of such preparations as are always, or at least preferably, made by weight (for instance, No. 2, Acidum Carbolicum Iodatum; No. 10, Boroglycerinum, etc., etc.), definite weights and measures have been used in the case of all those which are taken or administered by measure.

In the choice of the terms expressing the different denominations of weights and measures, some variation will be noticed, which is, however, introduced designedly. For instance, in No. 197 (Linimentum Opii Compositum), the first item is 1½ fluidounces; the second, 120 grains; the third, 4 fluidounces; the fourth, 180 minims; the fifth, 6 fluidounces, etc. The term "180 minims" was preferred to "3 fluidrachms," to break the monotony of the *fluid* terms, so as to diminish the risk of a mistake. And this method has been applied also in many other cases.

Regarding the nomenclature, the Committee has selected what appeared to them the most suitable and expressive titles. Probably many of the preparations in the work will never be ordered under their Latin names, as for instance, "Pulvis Hydrargyri Chloridi Mitis et Jalapæ" ("Calomel and Jalap"); yet it was deemed necessary to introduce such titles, in order to secure a homogeneous alphabetical arrangement.

In the selection of the particular process or working formula for each preparation, the Committee has proceeded with all the care that it was possible to bestow upon it. All suggestions, recommendations and criticisms were carefully and impartially considered, and, whenever possible, practically tested. It is not to be expected, however, that the Committee has always succeeded in making the best selection. Indeed, many of the formulæ will, no doubt, hereafter, require modification to make them more perfect, after a sufficient time has elapsed to fully test the merits of the different processes.

It was not within the province of the Committee to meddle with matters of which the medical practitioner or the therapeutist is the proper and competent judge. In most cases, it was sufficient to take a formula, just as it was already in existence, and to adopt it either entirely without change, or to restrict the modifications to the unessential features without affecting its therapeutic value, and merely with a view to improve its form. There are, however, a number of preparations in which more radical changes appeared desirable. In these cases the Committee availed itself of the advice of competent medical authorities, either by personal interviews or by correspondence.

The mission which this work is to fulfil can only be properly accomplished by the co-operation of the medical profession. It is, therefore, of the greatest importance that the members of this profession, throughout the country, be made acquainted with the existence, contents and objects of this book, and that, if the same be approved by them, as is confidently expected, they will consent to accept the preparations made in accordance with the formulæ contained therein, instead of designating any special maker's product.

In the execution of its task, the National Committee has been fortunate enough to avail itself of valuable advice and assistance, both voluntary and solicited, from many members of the profession and other sources. At the request of the Committee, the three Societies who had issued the pamphlet above spoken of, continued the several committees formerly appointed by them, and this increase of the working nucleus of the National Committee has been of the utmost importance to a successful termination of its allotted task, since without this assistance, it would have been physically impossible for it to perform the large number of experiments, and to prepare the many hundreds of specimens, necessary to decide on the merits of the various proposed formulæ. The gentlemen who have so generously assisted the Committee, and to whom special thanks are due, are: Messrs. Gustavus Balser, Julius Kalish, Edward L. Milhau, and Henry Schmid, from the College of Pharmacy of the City of New York; Messrs. Donald L. Cameron, Thomas D. McElhenie, J. P. Heyen, Louis E. Nicot, and Charles R. Paddock, of the Kings County Pharmaceutical Society; and Messrs. Theodore Louis, Charles E. P. Meumann, Gustavus Pfingsten, Gustavus Ramsperger, and Charles F. Schleussner, of the German Apothecaries' Society of the City of New York. Very valuable assistance has also been rendered to the Committee by the following gentlemen: Prof. Joseph P. Remington, Prof. J. M. Maisch, and Mr. Alfred B. Taylor of Philadelphia, Prof. J. U. Lloyd of Cincinnati, Dr. Robert G. Eccles of Brooklyn, Prof. Charles E. Munroe, U. S. N., of Newport,

R. I., Prof. Alfred M. Mayer of Hoboken, N. J., Messrs. Charles F. Heebner, W. M. Massey, and B. T. Fairchild of New York, Mr. O. A. A. Rouillion of Brooklyn, Mr. C. H. Bernhard of Madison, and Mr. A. Conrath of Milwaukee, Wis., Dr. Charles Mohr of Mobile, Ala., Mr. J. H. Dawson, and Prof. W. T. Wenzell of San Francisco, Messrs. R. B. Ferguson, W. S. Thompson, and G. G. C. Simms of Washington, D. C., Dr. A. B. Lyons of Detroit, Mich., Messrs. S. A. D. Sheppard, and J. W. Colcord of Boston, Mass., Mr. J. D. A. Hartz of College Point, N. Y., Mr. Albert E. Ebert, Prof. E. B. Stuart and Mr. Charles L. Feldkamp of Chicago, Ill., the Committees on Unofficinal Formulæ appointed by various State Pharmaceutical Associations during the last two years, and many others.

The Committee, on behalf of the American Pharmaceutical Association, now turns over its work to the public, and expresses the hope that it will be accepted as a standard and guide, whenever possible. In order that it may be rendered more perfect and complete, it is respectfully urged that any defects, omissions, or errors, be carefully noted, and that a list of these, as well as suggestions and propositions for a future revision, be sent to the Secretary of the American Pharmaceutical Association, or to any Formulary Committee that may hereafter be appointed.

THE COMMITTEE ON NATIONAL FORMULARY OF THE AMERICAN PHARMACEUTICAL ASSOCIATION.

MEMBERS AT LARGE, AND EDITING COMMITTEE.

Charles Rice, Chairman	New York, N. Y.
P. W. Bedford, Secretary	New York, N. Y.
S. J. Bendiner	New York, N. Y.
W. P. DeForest	Brooklyn, N. Y.
A. Tscheppe	New York, N. Y.

MEMBERS FROM PHARMACEUTICAL ASSOCIATIONS.

Alabama	P. C. Candidus, Mobile.
Arkansas	J. E. Gibson, Little Rock.
California	Emlen Painter, New York, N. Y.
Connecticut	C. A. Rapelye, Hartford.
Dist. Columbia	H. E. Kalusowski, Washington.
Dakota	H. L. Warne, Mitchell.
Georgia	J. W. Rankin, Atlanta.
Illinois	C. S. Hallberg, Chicago.
Indiana	G. W. Sloan, Indianapolis.
Iowa	T. W. Ruete, Dubuque.
Kansas	R. J. Brown, Leavenworth.
Kentucky	C. L. Diehl, Louisville.

Louisiana	A. K. Finlay, New Orleans.
Maryland	C. Caspari, jr., Baltimore.
Massachusetts	W. W. Bartlet, Boston.
Michigan	A. B. Stevens, Detroit.
Minnesota	W. S. Getty, St. Paul.
Mississippi	S. P. Head, Terry.
Missouri	J. M. Good, St. Louis.
Nebraska	N. A. Kuhn, Omaha.
New Hampshire	M. S. Woodman, West Lebanon.
New Jersey	Chas. B. Smith, Newark.
New York	L. F. Stevens, Brooklyn.
North Carolina	E. V. Zoeller, Tarboro.
Ohio	L. C. Hopp, Cleveland.
Pennsylvania	C. T. George, Harrisburg.
Rhode Island	E. A. Calder, Providence.
South Carolina	G. J. Luhn, Charleston.*
Tennessee	J. S. Robinson, Memphis.
Texas	E. M. Wells, Fort Worth.
Virginia	C. A. Santos, Norfolk.
West Virginia	C. Menkemeller, Wheeling.
Wisconsin	F. B. Power, Madison.
Ontario, Can	E. Gregory, Lindsay.
Quebec, Can.	W. Ahern, Quebec.

* Deceased.

ERRATA.

PAGE

8—Form. 22. Cordiale Rubi Fructus is preferably prepared thus: "Percolate the powdered spices with Diluted Alcohol to obtain *two* (2) *pints* of tincture, and add to this the *three* (3) *pints* of Blackberry Juice. Then add *one hundred and twenty* (120) *grains* of Purified Talcum, set the mixture aside for twelve hours, or longer, if convenient, occasionally shaking, and filter. To the filtrate add the Syrup."

18—Form. 51. At the end of the note printed in italics read: "*and 1 grain of Pepsin* (*N. F.*)"

28—Form. 83. Read: "Syrup . . 3 fluidounces," instead of "4 fluidounces."

48—Form. 133. Read: "Menstruum I: Alcohol 9 fluidounces, Water 5 fluidounces, Glycerin 2 fluidounces. Menstruum II: Alcohol 9 fluidounces, Water, 7 fluidounces."

58—Form. 178. Read: "Sugar, in very fine powder, . . 640 parts."

81—Form. 235. At the end of the directions add: "Finally filter."

Form. 237. Read: "add the Bicarbonate of Sodium in divided portions."

84—Form. 244. Add the synonym: *Lotio Hydrargyri Flava* (Brit. Pharm.).

Form. 245. Add the synonym: *Lotio Hydrargyri Nigra* (Brit. Pharm.).

97—Form. 278. Read: "then transfer the mass to a strainer of Canton flannel, and add to the filtrate an equal volume of Alcohol. Collect the precipitate, drain it, and free it by pressure from as much of the adherent liquid as possible. Then spread it on shallow trays, and dry it by exposure to warm air, at a temperature not exceeding 40° C. (104° F.). Triturate the dry product, in a mortar, with *four* (4) *times* its weight of pure benzin; transfer the mass to a dry filter, and when the liquid has passed below the surface of the powder, follow it with enough fresh benzin to displace the retained portion. Lastly dry the powder between bibulous paper."

98—Form. 279. Line 6 from below, read: "should remain" for "may remain."

112—Form. 322 II. Read: "but so that it will retain its crystalline character."

Form. 323. Read: "Sugar, in very fine powder . . 290 parts."

130—Form. 368. Lines 17 and 16 from below, read: "replacing from time to time any Water lost by evaporation, and cautiously adding small portions of the Soda solution, until the magma is entirely dissolved."

139—Form. 389. In the note printed in italics, read: "*contains about ⅓ grain.*"

148—Form. 411. The words in the text "cut into thin slices and carefully freed from any adhering fine powder" apply to the Rhubarb, *before* it is weighed.

154—Form. 428. Among the ingredients insert "Syrup . . 1½ fluidounces." In the text read: "then gradually add, while stirring, the Syrup, previously mixed with *ten* (10) *fluidounces* of Angelica Wine, and afterwards the Tincture of Citro-Chloride of Iron."

A few discrepancies in nomenclature were noticed too late to be corrected, such as: Form. 21, "Indian Hemp," for "Indian Cannabis." Form. 23 and 70, "Extract of Liquorice," for "Extract of Glycyrrhiza;" Form. 359 and elsewhere, "Irish Moss" for "Chondrus." Form. 258 and 389, "Resin of Guaiac," for "Guaiac."—Form. 351. "Syrupus Actææ Compositus," should have been made a synonym, and the chief title should be "Syrupus Cimicifugæ Compositus."

NATIONAL FORMULARY

OF

UNOFFICINAL PREPARATIONS.

---

1. ACETUM AROMATICUM.

Aromatic Vinegar.

Oil of Lavender	4 minims.
Oil of Rosemary	4 "
Oil of Juniper	4 "
Oil of Peppermint	4 "
Oil of Cinnamon (Cassia)	4 "
Oil of Lemon	8 "
Oil of Cloves	8 "
Alcohol	3 fluidounces.
Acetic Acid (U. S. P.)	3 "
Water . . . . . enough to make	16 "

Dissolve the Oils in the Alcohol, add the Acetic Acid, and lastly, enough Water to make *sixteen* (16) *fluidounces.* Warm the turbid mixture, during several hours, at a temperature not exceeding 70° C. (158° F.), taking care that it shall not suffer loss by evaporation. Then set it aside for a few days, occasionally agitating, and filter.

2. ACIDUM CARBOLICUM IODATUM.

Iodized Carbolic Acid.

Phenol Iodatum. Iodized Phenol.

Iodine, reduced to powder	20 parts.
Carbolic Acid	76 "
Glycerin	4 "

Introduce the Iodine into a flask, add the Carbolic Acid, previously melted, and the Glycerin, and digest the mixture at a gentle heat, frequently agitating, until the Iodine is dissolved.

Keep the product in glass-stoppered vials, in a dark place.

3. ACIDUM HYPOPHOSPHOROSUM DILUTUM.

Diluted Hypophosphorous Acid.

Hypophosphite of Potassium	208	parts.
Tartaric Acid	300	"
Distilled Water	588	"
Diluted Alcohol	600	"

Dissolve the Hypophosphite of Potassium in the Distilled Water, and the Tartaric Acid in the Diluted Alcohol. Mix the two solutions in a flask, cork the latter well, and put it aside in a cold place during twelve hours. Then carefully decant the liquid into a funnel, the neck of which contains a pellet of absorbent cotton, or, if necessary, pass the liquid through a filter, care being taken that it shall not suffer loss by evaporation. Weigh the filtrate, which contains *ten* (10) *per cent.* of hypophosphorous acid, in a tared capsule, and evaporate the alcohol by means of a water-bath, at a temperature not exceeding 60° C. (140° F.). Then allow the liquid to cool, and add enough Distilled Water to restore the original weight of the filtrate. Preserve the product in well-stoppered bottles.

Hypophosphorous Acid thus prepared contains 10 per cent. of absolute hypophosphorous acid (H_3PO_2), and has a specific gravity of 1.060 at 15° C. (59° F.) If the acid is required for immediate use, and the presence of alcohol is not objectionable, the mixture of the two solutions need be cooled only a short time, and the filtrate may be used at once. If a 50 per cent. acid is required, the concentration may be cautiously continued until the desired percentage has been attained. A 50 per cent. acid has a specific gravity of about 1.406 at 15° C. (59° F.)

4. ACIDUM METAPHOSPHORICUM DILUTUM.

Diluted Metaphosphoric Acid.

Acidum Phosphoricum Glaciale Dilutum. Diluted Glacial Phosphoric Acid.

Glacial Phosphoric Acid	780 grains.
Distilled Water	enough to make 16 fluidounces.

Dissolve the Acid in the Water, without heat.

This preparation should be kept in a cool and dark place, and should not be prepared in larger quantity than may be consumed within a few months.

Note.—The resulting product contains about 10 per cent. of metaphosphoric acid, provided the glacial acid was free from impurities. That which is sold in form of glassy lumps is usually of sufficient purity. The variety in form of round sticks is more or less impure, containing generally more than 15 per cent. of phosphate of sodium. If this variety is alone available, a proportionately larger quantity must be taken, to be determined, if time permits, by an assay of the free acid present. If no special accuracy is required, about 900 grains of this variety of the acid may be reckoned to be equivalent to the quantity directed in the above given formula.

Whenever Pyrophosphate of Iron (U. S. P.) forms one of the ingredients of a mixture containing Diluted Phosphoric Acid, the officinal tribasic acid is unsuitable, as it produces with the salt a gelatinous precipitate. If a clear mixture is required, the above preparation is to be used in place of the officinal. The same may be done when Phosphate of Iron (U. S. P.) is prescribed, though the precipitate caused by the officinal acid in this case is not as bulky, and under certain conditions may not form at all.

5. AQUA CHLOROFORMI.

Chloroform Water.

Purified Chloroform	30 minims.
Distilled Water	10 fluidounces.

Shake them together in a capacious bottle, until the Chloroform is dissolved, or until only a small quantity remains which cannot be dissolved by further agitation. Then filter in a covered funnel. Keep the product in well-stoppered bottles.

Note.—Chloroform water, aside from its medicinal properties, is an efficient preservative agent, and forms a good solvent, in place of water, for preparing solutions which require to be kept free from micro-organisms.

6. AQUA HAMAMELIDIS.

Hamamelis Water.

Witchhazel Water. Witchhazel Extract.

Hamamelis, shoots and twigs	10 pounds.
Water	20 pints.
Alcohol	1½ "

Place the Hamamelis in a still, add the Water and Alcohol, and allow the mixture to macerate during twenty-four hours. Distil *ten* (10) *pints* by applying direct heat, or preferably, by means of steam.

Note.—This preparation should be made only from the fresh young twigs of Hamamelis, which are collected for this purpose preferably, when the plant is in flower, in the late autumn of the year.

7. AQUA SEDATIVA.

Sedative Water.

Lotio Ammoniacalis Camphorata (Codex). *Eau Sédative de Raspail.*

Water of Ammonia	2 fluidounces.
Spirit of Camphor	90 minims.
Chloride of Sodium	1 troy ounce.
Water . . . . enough to make	16 fluidounces.

Dissolve the Chloride of Sodium in about *eight* (8) *fluidounces* of Water, add the Water of Ammonia and Spirit of Camphor, and finally enough Water to make *sixteen* (16) *fluidounces*.

Shake the liquid when it is to be dispensed.

19. COLLODIUM IODOFORMATUM.

Iodoform Collodion.

Iodoform	5 parts.
Flexible Collodion	95 "

Dissolve the Iodoform in the Flexible Collodion by agitation.

20. COLLODIUM TIGLII.

Croton Oil Collodion.

Croton Oil	10 parts.
Flexible Collodion	90 "

Mix them.

21. COLLODIUM SALICYLATUM COMPOSITUM.

Compound Salicylated Collodion.

Corn Collodion.

Salicylic Acid	11 parts.
Extract of Indian Hemp	2 "
Alcohol	10 "
Flexible Collodion . . . . enough to make	100 parts.

Dissolve the Extract of Indian Hemp in the Alcohol, and the Salicylic Acid in about *fifty* (50) *parts* of Flexible Collodion contained in a tared bottle. Then add the former solution to the latter, and finally add enough Flexible Collodion to make *one hundred* (100) *parts*.

22. CORDIALE RUBI FRUCTUS.

Blackberry Cordial.

Blackberry Juice	3 pints.
Cinnamon, in coarse powder	2 troy ounces.
Cloves, in coarse powder	½ troy ounce.
Nutmeg, in coarse powder	½ " "
Diluted Alcohol	2 pints.
Syrup	3 "

Digest the Spices with the Diluted Alcohol for eight days; then mix with the Blackberry Juice and strain; lastly, add the Syrup.

23. DECOCTUM ALOES COMPOSITUM.

Compound Decoction of Aloes.

Aqueous Extract of Aloes	120 grains.
Myrrh	90 "
Saffron	90 "
Carbonate of Potassium	60 "
Extract of Glycyrrhiza, in powder	1 troy ounce.
Compound Tincture of Cardamom	8 fluidounces.
Water . . . . enough to make	30 "

Reduce the Myrrh and Extract of Aloes to a coarse powder, mix this with the Carbonate of Potassium and Extract of Liquorice in a suitable covered vessel, and pour on *twenty* (20) *fluidounces* of Water; boil for five minutes, and add the Saffron. When cool, add the Compound Tincture of Cardamom, and allow the mixture to macerate for two hours; then filter through flannel, and add enough Water to make the product measure *thirty* (30) *fluidounces.*

This preparation should be freshly made when wanted for use.

24. ELIXIR ACIDI SALICYLICI.

Elixir of Salicylic Acid.

Salicylic Acid	640 grains.
Citrate of Potassium	2 troy ounces.
Glycerin	8 fluidounces.
Aromatic Elixir . . . enough to make	16 "

Dissolve the Citrate of Potassium in the Glycerin with the aid of a gentle heat. Add the Salicylic Acid, and continue the heat until it is dissolved. Then add enough Aromatic Elixir to make *sixteen* (16) *fluidounces.*

This Elixir should be freshly made when wanted for use.

Each fluidrachm contains 5 grains of Salicylic Acid.

25. ELIXIR ADJUVANS.

Adjuvant Elixir.

Sweet Orange Peel, recently dried	2 troy ounces.
Wild Cherry	4 " "
Glycyrrhiza, Russian, peeled	8 " "
Coriander	1 troy ounce.
Caraway	1 " "
Alcohol,	
Water	each, a sufficient quantity.
Syrup . . . enough to make	1 gallon.

Grind the Wild Cherry to a moderately coarse (No. 40) powder, moisten it with *four* (4) *fluidounces* of Water and set it aside for twelve hours. Reduce the other solids also to a moderately coarse (No. 40) powder, mix this intimately with the Wild Cherry, and having mixed *one* (1) *volume* of Alcohol with *two* (2) *volumes* of Water, moisten the powder with *four* (4) *fluidounces* of the mixture, and pack tightly in a percolator. Then gradually pour menstruum on top until *ninety-six* (96) *fluidounces* of percolate are obtained. Mix this with *thirty-two* (32) *fluidounces* of Syrup, and filter.

Note.—This preparation is chiefly intended as a vehicle, particularly for acrid or saline remedies.

93. ELIXIR QUININÆ ET PHOSPHATUM COMPOSITUM.

Compound Elixir of Quinine and Phosphates.

Sulphate of Quinine	32	grains.
Phosphate of Iron (U. S. P. 1880)	128	"
Citrate of Potassium	128	"
Syrup of Lactophosphate of Calcium	4	fluidounces.
Water	½	fluidounce.
Aromatic Elixir . . . enough to make	16	fluidounces.

Dissolve the Sulphate of Quinine in *ten* (10) *fluidounces* of Aromatic Elixir, if necessary with the aid of a gentle heat. Dissolve the Phosphate of Iron and the Citrate of Potassium in the Water, and add the solution to that first prepared. Then add the Syrup of Lactophosphate of Calcium, and lastly, enough Aromatic Elixir to make *sixteen* (16) *fluidounces*. Filter, if necessary.

Each fluidrachm contains ¼ grain of Sulphate of Quinine, 1 grain of Phosphate of Iron, and about ¾ grain of so-called Lactophosphate of Calcium.

94. ELIXIR QUININÆ VALERIANATIS ET STRYCHNINÆ.

Elixir of Valerianate of Quinine and Strychnine.

Valerianate of Quinine	128	grains.
Sulphate of Strychnine	1¼	"
Compound Tincture of Cudbear	120	minims.
Aromatic Elixir . . . enough to make	16	fluidounces.

Triturate the Valerianate of Quinine and the Sulphate of Strychnine with about *eight* (8) *fluidounces* of Aromatic Elixir, until they are dissolved. Then add the Compound Tincture of Cudbear, and lastly, enough Aromatic Elixir to make *sixteen* (16) *fluidounces*. Filter, if necessary.

Each fluidrachm contains 1 grain of Valerianate of Quinine and $\frac{1}{100}$ grain of Sulphate of Strychnine.

95. ELIXIR RHAMNI PURSHIANÆ.

Elixir of Rhamnus Purshiana.

Elixir of Cascara Sagrada.

Fluid Extract of Rhamnus Purshiana	4	fluidounces.
Elixir of Glycyrrhiza	4	"
Compound Elixir of Taraxacum	8	"

Mix them. Allow the mixture to stand a few days, if convenient, and filter.

Each fluidrachm represents 15 grains of Rhamnus Purshiana.

96. ELIXIR RHAMNI PURSHIANÆ COMPOSITUM.

Compound Elixir of Rhamnus Purshiana.

Compound Elixir of Cascara Sagrada. Elixir Laxativum; Elixir Purgans; Laxative Elixir.

Fluid Extract of Rhamnus Purshiana	2 fluidounces.
Fluid Extract of Senna	1¼ "
Fluid Extract of Juglans	1 fluidounce.
Fluid Extract of Glycyrrhiza	½ "
Compound Tincture of Cardamom	½ "
Aromatic Spirit	2 fluidounces.
Syrup	6 "
Purified Talcum	120 grains.
Water enough to make	16 fluidounces.

Mix the Fluid Extracts with the Compound Tincture of Cardamom and the Aromatic Spirit; then add the Syrup, and lastly, enough Water to make *sixteen* (16) *fluidounces.* Incorporate the Purified Talcum thoroughly with the mixture, and filter.

The average dose of this preparation, for an adult, is 1 to 2 teaspoonfuls.

97. ELIXIR RHEI.

Elixir of Rhubarb.

Sweet Tincture of Rhubarb (U. S. P.)	8 fluidounces.
Deodorized Alcohol	1 fluidounce.
Water	3 fluidounces.
Glycerin	2 "
Syrup	2 "

Mix them, and filter.

Each fluidrachm represents about 2¼ grains of Rhubarb.

98. ELIXIR RHEI ET MAGNESII ACETATIS.

Elixir of Rhubarb and Acetate of Magnesium.

Elixir Rhei et Magnesiæ. Elixir of Rhubarb and Magnesia.

Magnesia, calcined	144 grains.
Acetic Acid (U. S. P.)	a sufficient quantity.
Fluid Extract of Rhubarb	2 fluidounces.
Aromatic Elixir enough to make	16 fluidounces.

Dissolve the Magnesia in *two and one-half* (2½) *fluidounces* of Acetic Acid, with the aid of a gentle heat, adding, if necessary, a little more Acetic Acid, drop by drop, until the solution is neutral to test-paper. Then add the Fluid Extract and enough Aromatic Elixir to make *sixteen* (16) *fluidounces*, and filter.

Each fluidrachm represents about 4 grains of Acetate of Magnesium and 7½ grains of Rhubarb.

117. EMULSIO OLEI MORRHUÆ CUM CALCII PHOSPHATE.

Emulsion of Cod-Liver Oil with Phosphate of Calcium.

Emulsion of Cod-Liver Oil with Phosphate of Lime.

Cod-Liver Oil	8 fluidounces.
Mucilage of Irish Moss (N. F.)	5 "
Phosphate of Calcium	256 grains.
Syrup of Tolu	1 fluidounce.
Alcohol	1 "
Flavoring	a sufficient quantity.
Water	enough to make 16 fluidounces.

To the Mucilage of Irish Moss, contained in a suitable vessel, gradually add the Cod-Liver Oil and prepare an emulsion as directed under *Emulsio Olei Morrhuæ.* Triturate the Phosphate of Calcium with the Syrup of Tolu and add this to the emulsion; then add the Alcohol, Flavoring, and enough Water to make *sixteen* (16) *fluidounces.* Mix the whole thoroughly together.

Note.—If any other method of emulsifying the oil is adopted, the Phosphate of Calcium should be triturated with Water, or some other of the liquid constituents, which are added last.

118. EMULSIO OLEI MORRHUÆ CUM EXTRACTO MALTI.

Emulsion of Cod-Liver Oil with Extract of Malt.

Cod-Liver Oil	8 fluidounces.
Mucilage of Dextrin (N. F.)	2 "
Extract of Malt	6 "

To the Mucilage of Dextrin contained in a suitable bottle, add the Extract of Malt, and mix them thoroughly by agitation. Then gradually add the Cod-Liver Oil, first in small portions, agitating each time until the last-added portion is perfectly incorporated.

Note.—Extract of Malt, most suitable for this preparation, should have about the same consistence as Balsam of Peru, at a temperature of 15° C. (59° F.)

119. EMULSIO OLEI MORRHUÆ CUM HYPOPHOSPHITE.

Emulsion of Cod-Liver Oil with Hypophosphite.

Cod-Liver Oil	8 fluidounces.
Mucilage of Irish Moss (N. F.)	5 "
Any Soluble Hypophosphite	128 grains.
Syrup of Tolu	1 fluidounce.
Alcohol	1 "
Flavoring	a sufficient quantity.
Water	enough to make 16 fluidounces.

Dissolve the Hypophosphite in the Mucilage of Irish Moss, and emulsify the Cod-Liver Oil with the latter as directed under *Emulsio Olei Morrhuæ*. Then add the Syrup of Tolu, Alcohol, and Flavoring, and finally, enough Water to make *sixteen* (16) *fluidounces*. Mix the whole thoroughly together.

Note.—If another method of emulsifying the oil is adopted, the Hypophosphite should be dissolved in the aqueous portion of the mixture.

If more than one Hypophosphite is directed in combination with Emulsion of Cod-Liver Oil, and no definite quantities of the salts are prescribed, equal parts of the several Hypophosphites may be taken, amounting altogether to 128 grains, for every pint of emulsion.

120. EMULSIO OLEI MORRHUÆ CUM PRUNO VIRGINIANA.

Emulsion of Cod-Liver Oil with Wild Cherry.

Cod-Liver Oil	8 fluidounces.
Mucilage of Irish Moss (N. F.)	5 "
Fluid Extract of Wild Cherry	1 fluidounce.
Syrup of Tolu	1 "
Alcohol	½ "
Flavoring	a sufficient quantity.
Water	enough to make 16 fluidounces.

To the Mucilage of Irish Moss, contained in a suitable bottle, gradually add the Cod-Liver Oil, and prepare an emulsion as directed under *Emulsio Olei Morrhuæ*. Next add the Fluid Extract of Wild Cherry, then the Syrup of Tolu, Alcohol, Flavoring, and enough Water to make *sixteen* (16) *fluidounces*.

Note.—If another method of emulsifying the oil is adopted, the Fluid Extract of Wild Cherry is to be added after the emulsion of the oil is accomplished, if necessary, with omission of a corresponding volume of one of the secondary constituents.

121. EMULSIO OLEI RICINI.

Emulsion of Castor Oil.

I. Irish Moss Emulsion of Castor Oil.

Castor Oil	5 fluidounces.
Mucilage of Irish Moss (N. F.)	5 "
Tincture of Vanilla	180 minims.
Syrup	3 fluidounces.
Water	enough to make 16 fluidounces.

To the Mucilage of Irish Moss, contained in a suitable bottle, add the Castor Oil in divided portions, agitating each time until the last-added portion has been emulsified. Then add the Tincture of Vanilla, the Syrup, and enough Water to make *sixteen* (16) *fluidounces*. Finally, mix the whole thoroughly together.

This emulsion should not be prepared in larger quantity than may be consumed within a short time.

Emulsion of Castor Oil may also be prepared by other methods capable of emulsifying the oil, provided the vehicles and ingredients are compatible with the therapeutic employment of the preparation. In absence of any specific directions of the prescriber, it is recommended that Castor Oil Emulsion be only prepared either by means of Irish Moss, or by means of Acacia.

II. Acacia Emulsion of Castor Oil.

Castor Oil	5 fluidounces.
Acacia, in fine powder	1½ troy ounces.
Tincture of Vanilla	180 minims.
Syrup	3 fluidounces.
Water . . . . enough to make	16 "

Mix the Syrup with *two* (2) *fluidounces* of Water, and triturate the Acacia with the mixture to a smooth paste. Then gradually incorporate with it the Castor Oil. Transfer the mixture to a bottle, add the Tincture of Vanilla, and enough Water to make *sixteen* (16) *fluidounces*. Finally, mix the whole thoroughly together.

This Emulsion should not be prepared in larger quantity than may be consumed within a short time.

122. EMULSIO OLEI TEREBINTHINÆ.

Emulsion of Oil of Turpentine.

Oil of Turpentine	½ fluidounce.
Acacia, in fine powder	30 grains.
Yolk of Egg	one (1)
Aromatic Elixir	½ fluidounce.
Cinnamon Water . . . . enough to make	4 fluidounces.

Triturate the Acacia with the Yolk of Egg, then add the Oil of Turpentine very slowly, continuing the trituration, and finally, add the Water and Aromatic Elixir in the same manner.

Emulsion of Oil of Turpentine, or of any *Volatile Oil*, may also be prepared according to the following general formula:

Volatile Oil	½ fluidounce.
Acacia, in fine powder	120 grains.
Syrup	1 fluidounce.
Water . . . . enough to make	4 fluidounces.

Pour the Volatile Oil into a dry four-ounce bottle, and, having corked the latter, agitate it so that the inner surface may be completely wetted by the Oil. Then add the Acacia, and shake again. Finally add the Syrup, and enough Water to make *four* (4) *fluidounces*, and mix thoroughly by shaking.

Note.—If this general formula is applied to Emulsion of Oil of Turpentine, and a product similar to that obtained by the first formula is desired, the Syrup should be replaced by Aromatic Elixir, and the Water by Cinnamon Water.

If a so-called "Emulsion" of a Volatile Oil is to be made more permanent, this may be accomplished by incorporating with it a small proportion of some bland fixed oil, such as Expressed Oil of Almond. Usually, 1 volume of the fixed oil will be sufficient for 2 volumes of the volatile oil.

In this case, the mixture should be made in a mortar, by trituration.

123. EMULSIO PHOSPHATICA.

Phosphatic Emulsion.

Mistura Phosphatica.

Cod-Liver Oil	4	fluidounces.
Glycerite of Yolk of Egg (U. S. P.)	2½	troy ounces.
Diluted Phosphoric Acid	360	minims.
Oil of Bitter Almond	10	"
Rum, Jamaica	4	fluidounces.
Orange Flower Water . . . . enough to make	16	fluidounces.

To the Glycerite of Yolk of Egg (Glyconin) contained in a suitable bottle, gradually add the Cod-Liver Oil, in small portions at a time, shaking after each addition, until the added portion is emulsified. Then gradually add the Phosphoric Acid, Rum, and Oil of Bitter Almond, incorporating them thoroughly. Finally, add enough Orange Flower Water to make *sixteen* (16) *fluidounces*, and mix the whole thoroughly.

124. EXTRACTA FLUIDA.

Fluid Extracts.

The Fluid Extracts for which formulæ are given in this Formulary, are intended to be of such a strength that *one* (1) *minim* shall represent *one* (1) *grain* of the air-dry, powdered drug.

Note.—The U. S. Pharm. directs that 100 cubic centimeters of fluid extract shall be obtained from 100 grammes of drug. Fluid extracts prepared in this ratio are 5 per cent. weaker than those which are made minim for grain. The difference between the two kinds is not regarded as being of material importance.

General Processes. The Fluid Extracts of this Formulary are to be prepared according to one of the following two general processes, the particular one to be employed being designated in each case.

Process A. The Menstruum contains no Glycerin.

Moisten *sixteen* (16) *troy ounces* of the drug with a sufficient quantity of the prescribed menstruum to render it distinctly damp and to maintain it so after several hours' maceration in a well covered vessel. When the drug has ceased to swell, pack it in a suitable percolator, pour a sufficient quantity of the menstruum on top, and, when the percolate begins to drop from the orifice, close the latter, cover the percolator, and allow the contents to macerate for twenty-four hours. Then permit the percolation to proceed. Receive the first *fourteen* (14) *fluidounces* of the percolate separately and set it aside. Then continue the percolation with the same menstruum until the drug is practically exhausted. Evaporate this second portion—at a temperature sufficiently low to prevent the loss of any important volatile constituent—to a soft extract, and dissolve this in a sufficient quantity of the menstruum so that when this is added to the reserved portion, the product will measure *sixteen* (16) *fluidounces*. Allow the Fluid Extract to stand a few days, or longer, if convenient, and filter, if necessary.

Process B. The Menstruum contains Glycerin.

Moisten *sixteen* (16) *troy ounces* of the drug with a sufficient quantity of Menstruum I (see note) to render it distinctly damp and to maintain it so after several hours' maceration in a well covered vessel. When the drug has ceased to swell, pack it in a suitable percolator and pour the remainder of Menstruum I on top. When this has just disappeared from the surface, follow it by a sufficient quantity of Menstruum II. As soon as the percolate begins to drop from the orifice, close the latter, cover the percolator, and allow the contents to macerate during twenty-four hours. Then permit the percolation to proceed. Receive the first *fourteen* (14) *fluidounces* of the percolate separately and set it aside. Then continue the percolation with Menstruum II, until the drug is practically exhausted. Evaporate this second portion—at a temperature sufficiently low to prevent the loss of any important volatile constituent—to a soft extract, and dissolve this in a sufficient quantity of Menstruum II, so that when this is added to the reserved portion, the product will measure *sixteen* (16) *fluidounces*. Allow the Fluid Extract to stand a few days, or longer, if convenient, and filter, if necessary.

Note.—"Menstruum I" and "Menstruum II" denote the several liquids which will be directed for preparing certain Fluid Extracts. Compare, for instance, Nos. 138, 140, 141.

When it is desired to avoid the use of heat in the preparation of any Fluid Extract, a method of *Fractional Percolation* may be employed, for which directions are given below.

This method involves the use of only *one* kind of menstruum, even in the case of drugs for which two different successive menstrua (I and II) are prescribed in this Formulary. In the case of the latter, a sufficient quantity of Menstruum I should be prepared to serve throughout the process.

Fractional Percolation.—Take of the drug, in powder of the prescribed fineness, *sixteen* (16) *troy ounces*, and divide this into three portions, of *eight* (8), *five* (5) and *three* (3) *troy ounces*, respectively.

Moisten the *first portion* (8 troy ounces) with the menstruum and percolate in the usual manner. Set aside the first *three* (3) *fluidounces* of the percolate, and continue until *twenty-four* (24) *fluidounces* more of percolate have passed, which should be received in several portions, so that the more concentrated will be separate from the last, weak percolate.

Then moisten the *second portion* of the drug (5 troy ounces) with the most concentrated of the percolates received during the preceding operation after the first 3 fluidounces had passed, and percolate again in the usual manner, using the several reserved percolates, successively, as menstrua. Set aside the first *five* (5) *fluidounces*, and continue the percolation until *ten* (10) *fluidounces* more have passed, which should also be received in several portions.

Finally moisten the *third portion* of the drug (3 troy ounces) with the most concentrated of the last reserved percolates, and proceed as directed for the second portion. Collect the first *eight* (8) *fluidounces* separately, and mix them with the two portions previously set aside so as to make *sixteen* (16) *fluidounces* of Fluid Extract.

125. EXTRACTUM ADONIDIS FLUIDUM.

Fluid Extract of Adonis.

From the root of *Adonis vernalis* Linné (Bird's Eye).

Process A (see No. 124).—No. 60 powder.
Menstruum: Alcohol.

126. EXTRACTUM ALETRIDIS FLUIDUM.

Fluid Extract of Aletris.

From the rhizome of *Aletris farinosa* Linné (Stargrass).

Process A (see No. 124).—No. 60 powder.
Menstruum: Diluted Alcohol.

127. EXTRACTUM ANGELICÆ RADICIS FLUIDUM.

Fluid Extract of Angelica Root.

From the root of *Angelica Archangelica* Linné (Angelica).

Process A (see No. 124).—No. 60 powder.
Menstruum: Alcohol, 3 volumes.
Water, 2 volumes.

128. EXTRACTUM APII GRAVEOLENTIS FLUIDUM.

Fluid Extract of Celery.

From the seed of *Apium graveolens* Linné (Celery).

Process A (see No. 124).—No. 60 powder.
Menstruum: Alcohol, 2 volumes.
Water, 1 volume.

294. PILULÆ COLOCYNTHIDIS ET PODOPHYLLI.

Pills of Colocynth and Podophyllum.

	Each pill contains:
Compound Extract of Colocynth	2½ grains.
Resin of Podophyllum	¼ grain.

295. PILULÆ FERRI CARBONATIS.

Pills of Carbonate of Iron.

Ferruginous Pills. Blaud's Pills. Chalybeate Pills.

Sulphate of Iron, in clear crystals	240 grains.
Carbonate of Potassium	140 "
Sugar	48 "
Tragacanth, in fine powder	16 "
Glycerin	10 minims.
Water	a sufficient quantity.

Triturate the Sulphate of Iron with the Sugar to a uniform powder. In another mortar triturate the Carbonate of Potassium with the Glycerin and *ten* (10) *minims* of Water. Add to this mixture the previously prepared powder, and beat the mass thoroughly until it assumes a greenish color. When the reaction appears to have terminated, incorporate the Tragacanth, and, if necessary, add a little more Water, so as to obtain a mass of a pilular consistence. Divide this into *ninety-six* (96) *pills*.

Each pill represents about 1 grain of Carbonate of Iron (ferrous).

Note.—Sometimes so-called "3 grain" Blaud's Pills (*Pilulæ Blaudii minores*) are prescribed or demanded. These may be prepared by using the quantities given in the above formula, and dividing the mass into *one hundred and sixty-eight* (168) *pills*.

296. PILULÆ GLONOINI.

Pills of Glonoin.

Pills of Nitroglycerin.

Spirit of Glonoin (N. F., 1%)	200 grains.
Althæa, in fine powder	198 "
Confection of Rose	a sufficient quantity.

Mix the Spirit of Glonoin intimately with the powdered Althæa, expose the mixture for a short time to the air, so that the alcohol may evaporate, then make a pill-mass by means of Confection of Rose, and divide it into *two hundred* (200) *pills*.

Each pill contains $\frac{1}{100}$ grain of Glonoin (Nitroglycerin).

297. PILULÆ LAXATIVÆ POST PARTUM.

Laxative Pills after Confinement.

Barker's Post Partum Pills.

	Each pill contains:
Compound Extract of Colocynth	$1\frac{2}{3}$ grains.
Aloes	$\frac{5}{6}$ grain.
Extract of Nux Vomica	$\frac{5}{12}$ "
Resin of Podophyllum	$\frac{1}{12}$ "
Ipecac, in fine powder	$\frac{1}{12}$ "
Extract of Hyoscyamus	$1\frac{1}{4}$ "

Note.—This is the formula generally employed by Dr. Fordyce Barker, except where special circumstances render modifications necessary. The formula usually quoted in manufacturers' lists and some formularies is not correct.

298. PILULÆ METALLORUM.

Metallic Pills.

Pilulæ Metallorum Amaræ. Bitter Metallic Pills.

	Each pill contains:
Reduced Iron	1 grain.
Sulphate of Quinine	1 "
Strychnine, alkaloid	$\frac{1}{20}$ "
Arsenious Acid	$\frac{1}{20}$ "

Note.—A similar combination is known under the name of *Aitken's Tonic Pills:*

	Each pill contains:
Reduced Iron	$\frac{2}{3}$ grain.
Sulphate of Quinine	1 "
Strychnine, alkaloid	$\frac{1}{50}$ "
Arsenious Acid	$\frac{1}{50}$ "

299. PILULÆ OPII ET CAMPHORÆ.

Pills of Opium and Camphor.

	Each pill contains:
Powdered Opium	1 grain.
Camphor	2 grains.

300. PILULÆ OPII ET PLUMBI.

Pills of Opium and Lead.

	Each pill contains:
Powdered Opium	1 grain.
Acetate of Lead	1 "

376. SYRUPUS PECTORALIS.

Pectoral Syrup.

Jackson's Pectoral (or *Cough*) *Syrup.*

Hydrochlorate of Morphine	4 grains.
Oil of Sassafras	4 minims.
Syrup of Acacia . . . . enough to make	16 fluidounces.

Dissolve the Hydrochlorate of Morphine in about *one* (1) *fluidounce* of the Syrup, add the Oil of Sassafras, and enough Syrup to make *sixteen* (16) *fluidounces.*

Each fluidrachm contains $\frac{1}{32}$ grain of Hydrochlorate of Morphine.

Note.—The original formula of Dr. Samuel Jackson's Cough Syrup was as follows: Sassafras Pith, 60 grains; Acacia, 1 ounce; Sugar, 28 av. ounces; Muriate of Morphine, 8 grains; Water, enough to make 32 fluidounces. The Sassafras Pith was afterwards uniformly replaced by Oil of Sassafras, and the other constituents of the Syrup have been more or less altered, so that a number of different formulæ are in vogue in different sections of the country. It is recommended that the above be followed, if possible, for the sake of uniformity. (See Note to No. 373).

377. SYRUPUS PHOSPHATUM COMPOSITUS.

Compound Syrup of the Phosphates.

Chemical Food.

Precipitated Carbonate of Calcium	256 grains.
Phosphate of Iron (U. S. P. 1880)	128 "
Phosphate of Ammonium	128 "
Bicarbonate of Potassium	32 "
Bicarbonate of Sodium	32 "
Citric Acid	1 troy ounce.
Glycerin	1 fluidounce.
Phosphoric Acid (50 %)	2 fluidounces.
Orange Flower Water	2 "
Tincture of Cudbear (N. F.)	120 minims.
Sugar	8 troy ounces.
Water . . . . enough to make	16 fluidounces.

Triturate the Precipitated Carbonate of Calcium with the Bicarbonate of Potassium and Sodium, the Citric Acid, Glycerin, and Orange Flower Water, and gradually add the Phosphoric Acid, stirring until solution has been effected. Dissolve the Phosphate of Iron and the Phosphate of Ammonium in *four* (4) *fluidounces* of hot Water, cool, and add the solution to that previously prepared. Filter the whole through a pellet of absorbent cotton placed in the neck of a funnel, and receive the filtrate in a graduated bottle containing the Sugar. Agitate until the latter is dissolved, then add the Tincture of Cudbear, and lastly, enough Water to make *sixteen* (16) *fluidounces.*

Each fluidrachm contains about 2 grains of Phosphate of Calcium, 1 grain, each, of the Phosphates of Iron and of Ammonium, and smaller quantities of the Phosphates of Potassium and Sodium.

378. SYRUPUS RHAMNI CATHARTICÆ.

Syrup of Rhamnus Cathartica.

Syrup of Buckthorn Berries. Syrupus Spinæ Cervinæ.

Sugar	13 troy ounces.
Fermented Juice of Buckthorn Berries,	enough to make 16 fluidounces.

Dissolve the Sugar in *seven* (7) *fluidounces* of the Juice, with the aid of a gentle heat, allow the Syrup to cool, then add enough of the Juice to make *sixteen* (16) *fluidounces*, and strain, if necessary.

Note.—This preparation is practically identical with that officinal in the *Germ. Pharm.* The species of Buckthorn to be used is the *Rhamnus cathartica* Linné, native of Europe, and naturalized, to some extent, in the U. S. If the fresh berries cannot be obtained, the imported fermented juice may be used in preparing the Syrup.

379. SYRUPUS RUBI AROMATICUS.

Aromatic Syrup of Blackberry.

Rubus (U. S. P.)	2 troy ounces.
Cinnamon	120 grains.
Nutmeg	120 "
Cloves	60 "
Allspice	60 "
Diluted Alcohol	a sufficient quantity.
Sugar	10 troy ounces.
Blackberry Juice	a sufficient quantity.

Reduce the Rubus (Blackberry Root) and the Aromatics to a moderately coarse (No. 40) powder, and percolate it, in the usual manner, with the Diluted Alcohol, until *four* (4) *fluidounces* of percolate are obtained. To this add *seven* (7) *fluidounces* of Blackberry Juice, and dissolve the Sugar in the liquid by agitation. Lastly, add enough Blackberry Juice to make *sixteen* (16) *fluidounces.*

380. SYRUPUS SANGUINARIÆ.

Syrup of Sanguinaria.

Syrup of Bloodroot.

Sanguinaria, in No. 20 powder	$3\frac{1}{2}$ troy ounces.
Acetic Acid	2 fluidounces.
Sugar	13 troy ounces.
Water	enough to make 16 fluidounces.

Mix the Acetic Acid with *six* (6) *fluidounces* of Water, moisten the Sanguinaria with a sufficient quantity of this menstruum, and allow it to macerate for two hours. Then pack it in a glass percolator, and percolate in the usual manner, first with the remainder of the menstruum previously prepared, and afterwards with Water until *twelve* (12) *fluidounces* of percolate are obtained, or until the Sanguinaria is practically exhausted. Evaporate the percolate, at a moderate heat, to *seven* (7) *fluidounces*. In this dissolve the Sugar with a gentle heat, if necessary, and add enough Water to make *sixteen* (16) *fluidounces*.

Each fluidrachm represents about 13 grains of Sanguinaria.

381. SYRUPUS SENNÆ AROMATICUS.

Aromatic Syrup of Senna.

Senna	2 troy ounces.
Jalap	384 grains.
Rhubarb	128 "
Cinnamon	30 "
Cloves	30 "
Nútmeg	15 "
Oil of Lemon	10 minims.
Sugar	12 troy ounces.
Diluted Alcohol	enough to make 16 fluidounces.

Reduce the drugs to a moderately fine (No. 50) powder, add to it the Oil of Lemon, and percolate it, in the usual manner, with Diluted Alcohol. Remove the first *eight* (8) *fluidounces* of the percolate, and dissolve in this the Sugar, with the aid of a gentle heat, if necessary, but avoiding loss of alcohol by evaporation. Allow the solution to cool, collect a further portion of percolate, and add it to the Syrup, so as to make *sixteen* (16) *fluidounces*.

Each fluidrachm represents 7½ grains of Senna, 3 grains of Jalap, and 1 grain of Rhubarb, with aromatics.

382. SYRUPUS SENNÆ COMPOSITUS.

Compound Syrup of Senna.

Fluid Extract of Senna	1024 minims.
Fluid Extract of Rhubarb	256 "
Fluid Extract of Frangula	256 "
Oil of Gaultheria	30 "
Alcohol	1 fluidounce.
Syrup	enough to make 16 fluidounces.

Dissolve the Oil of Gaultheria in the Alcohol, and add this to the mixed Fluid Extracts. Then add enough Syrup to make *sixteen* (16) *fluidounces*, and mix by agitation.

Each fluidrachm represents 8 grains of Senna, 2 grains of Rhubarb, and 2 grains of Frangula.

383. SYRUPUS SODII HYPOPHOSPHITIS.

Syrup of Hypophosphite of Sodium.

Hypophosphite of Sodium	256 grains.
Citric Acid	10 "
Sugar	12 troy ounces.
Water	enough to make 16 fluidounces.

Dissolve the Hypophosphite of Sodium and the Citric Acid in *eight* (8) *fluidounces* of Water, and filter the solution. In this dissolve the Sugar by agitation, and pass enough Water through the filter, to make the product measure *sixteen* (16) *fluidounces.*

Each fluidrachm contains 2 grains of Hypophosphite of Sodium.

384. SYRUPUS STILLINGIÆ COMPOSITUS.

Compound Syrup of Stillingia.

Compound Fluid Extract of Stillingia (N. F.)	4 fluidounces.
Purified Talcum	120 grains.
Sugar	11 troy ounces.
Water	enough to make 16 fluidounces.

Mix the Compound Fluid Extract of Stillingia with the Purified Talcum, and afterwards with *four and one-half* (4½) *fluidounces* of Water, and shake them together thoroughly. Then pour the mixture upon a wetted filter, add the Sugar to the filtrate, and pass enough Water through the filter to make the product, after the Sugar has been dissolved by agitation, measure *sixteen* (16) *fluidounces.*

Each fluidrachm represents 15 minims of Compound Fluid Extract of Stillingia (see No. 170).

385. TALCUM PURIFICATUM.

Purified Talcum.

Talcum, in fine powder	100 parts.
Hydrochloric Acid	15 "
Water	a sufficient quantity.

Mix *five hundred* (500) *parts* of boiling Water with the Talcum, gradually add *ten* (10) *parts* of the Hydrochloric Acid, and boil the mixture during fifteen minutes. Then allow the suspended Talcum to subside, pour off the supernatant liquid, and boil the residue again with *five hundred* (500) *parts* of Water mixed with the remainder of the Hydrochloric Acid. Again allow the mixture to become clear by settling, pour off the supernatant liquid, and wash the residue with Water, by repeated decantation, until a portion of the wash-water, filtered and placed in a test-tube, ceases to produce a precipitate with test-solution of nitrate of silver acidified with nitric acid. Then transfer the magma to a close linen or muslin strainer, allow it to drain, and dry it by heat.

Note.—Purified Talcum is used as an aid in filtering turbid liquids containing finely-divided matters in suspension, which are apt to pass through the filter, or to stop up its pores.

386. TINCTURÆ.

Tinctures.

General Process.—All Tinctures, for which no working formula is provided by the U. S. Pharmacopœia, the National Formulary, or some other work of authority, and the strength of which is not otherwise specified by the prescriber, should be prepared in the following proportions:

The Drug, properly comminuted	2 troy ounces.
The Menstruum . . . . enough to make	16 fluidounces.

Note.—The choice of the menstruum will depend upon the nature of the drug, and in some cases upon the uses to which the Tincture is to be applied. In general, it may be stated that, if the useful constituents are soluble in alcohol, and but slightly, or not at all soluble in water, strong alcohol should be used as a menstruum. Whenever it is possible, and consistent with the intended use of the preparation, the alcoholic strength of the menstruum should be made to approach that of Diluted Alcohol, the object being not only to exhaust the Drug of all its useful constituents, but also to retain them in solution.

If the drug is fibrous and can be dried and powdered without injury or loss of useful constituents, percolation is preferable. If the drug is resinous and partly, or almost wholly soluble in the menstruum, or if it is fibrous, and cannot well be powdered without undergoing injury, maceration should be resorted to. In the latter case, the drug, comminuted as much as possible, should be kept in contact with the full quantity of the menstruum for two weeks, or until the soluble matters are extracted, the liquid portion strained off, and the remainder of the tincture contained in the residue on the strainer carefully displaced by washing with a fresh portion of the menstruum until 16 fluidounces of tincture are obtained for every 2 troy ounces of drug used in the operation.

The preparation of Tinctures from Fluid Extracts, instead of from the original drugs themselves, is not recommended. In some special cases, however, when the crude drug is not accessible, or when a tincture, which is not at hand and otherwise unobtainable, is required for immediate use, it may be prepared, extemporaneously, from the corresponding fluid extract, provided that the latter is known to fully represent the active constituents of the drug which are intended to be contained in the tincture (see formulas 387, 411, 412).

387. TINCTURA ACONITI, FLEMING.

Fleming's Tincture of Aconite.

1. **Aconite** (root), in fine powder	10 troy ounces.
Alcohol . . . . enough to make	15 fluidounces.

Moisten the Aconite with enough Alcohol to render it distinctly damp and to maintain it so after twenty-four hours' maceration in a well covered vessel. Then pack it tightly in a percolator, and percolate it slowly, in the usual manner, with Alcohol, until *fifteen* (15) *fluidounces* of tincture are obtained.

Note.—This preparation is still prescribed by many physicians. It is recommended that their attention be directed to the officinal Fluid Extract and Tincture of Aconite, so that the above preparation may be gradually abandoned.

When this preparation is required for immediate use, and it is not otherwise available, it may be prepared in the following manner (see Note to No. 386):

2. Fluid Extract of Aconite	10	fluidounces.
Alcohol	5	"

Mix them.

388. TINCTURA AMARA.

Bitter Tincture.

Stomachic Tincture. Bitter Stomachic Drops. Stomach Drops.

Gentian	384	grains.
Centaury, herb	384	"
Bitter Orange Peel	256	"
Orange Berries	128	"
Zedoary, root	128	"
Alcohol,		
Water, each	enough to make 16	fluidounces.

Reduce the drugs to a moderately coarse (No. 40) powder, and percolate it, in the usual manner, with a mixture of *two* (2) *volumes* of Alcohol and *one* (1) *volume* of Water, until *sixteen* (16) *fluidounces* of percolate are obtained.

Note.—Centaury is the herb of *Erythræa Centaurium* Persoon. Orange Berries are the unripe fruit of *Citrus vulgaris* Risso, collected while small. Zedoary is the rhizome of *Curcuma Zedoaria* Roscoe. The product obtained by the above formula is practically identical with that which is officinal in the Germ. Pharm.

389. TINCTURA ANTACRIDA.

Antacrid Tincture.

Dysmenorrhœa Mixture. Fenner's Guaiac Mixture.

Corrosive Chloride of Mercury	40	grains.
Resin of Guaiac, in fine powder	2	troy ounces.
Canada Turpentine	2	" "
Oil of Sassafras	½	fluidounce.
Alcohol	enough to make 16	fluidounces.

Introduce the Resin of Guaiac and the Canada Turpentine into a flask, together with *twelve* (12) *fluidounces* of Alcohol, cork the flask loosely, and heat the contents, on a water-bath, slowly to boiling. Then cool the flask, and filter the contents through a small filter. Dissolve the Corrosive Chloride of Mercury in *one-half* (½) *fluidounce* of Alcohol, and add this solution, as well as the Oil of Sassafras, to the filtrate. Lastly, pass enough Alcohol through the filter to make the product measure *sixteen* (16) *fluidounces.*

Each fluidrachm contains nearly ⅓ grain of Corrosive Chloride of Mercury.

Note.—The dose of this preparation is about 10 to 20 minims.

427. VINUM CARNIS ET FERRI.

Wine of Beef and Iron.

Beef, Wine and Iron.

Extract of Beef	256 grains.
Tincture of Citro-Chloride of Iron	256 minims.
Hot Water	1 fluidounce.
Sherry Wine . . . . enough to make	16 fluidounces.

Pour the Hot Water upon the Extract of Beef contained in a mortar or other suitable vessel, and triturate until a smooth mixture results. Then gradually add, while stirring, *twelve* (12) *fluidounces* of Sherry Wine. Next add the Tincture and enough Sherry Wine to make *sixteen* (16) *fluidounees.* Transfer the mixture to a bottle, set this aside for a few days in a cold place, if convenient, filter, and pass enough Sherry Wine through the filter to restore the original volume.

Each fluidrachm represents 2 grains of Extract of Beef, and 2 minims of Tincture of Citro-Chloride of Iron.

Note.—Regarding Extract of Beef, see Note to No. 426.

428. VINUM CARNIS, FERRI ET CINCHONÆ.

Wine of Beef, Iron and Cinchona.

Beef, Wine, Iron and Cinchona.

Extract of Beef	256 grains.
Tincture of Citro-Chloride of Iron	256 minims.
Sulphate of Quinine	16 grains.
Sulphate of Cinchonidine	8 "
Citric Acid	6 "
Hot Water	1 fluidounce.
Angelica Wine . . . . enough to make	16 fluidounces.

Dissolve the Citric Acid and the Sulphates of Quinine and Cinchonidine in the Hot Water, and pour the solution upon the Extract of Beef contained in a mortar, or other suitable vessel. Triturate the liquid with the Extract, until they form a smooth mixture, then gradually add, while stirring, *twelve* (12) *fluidounces* of Angelica Wine, and afterwards the Tincture of Citro-Chloride of Iron. Transfer the mixture to a bottle, set this aside for a few days in a cold place, if convenient, filter, and pass enough Angelica Wine through the filter to make *sixteen* (16) *fluidounces.*

Each fluidrachm represents 2 grains of Extract of Beef, 2 minims of Tincture of Citro-Chloride of Iron, and small quantities of Cinchona alkaloids.

Note.—Regarding Extract of Beef, see Note to No. 426. Angelica Wine is a variety of sweet California wine.

429. VINUM ERYTHROXYLI.

Wine of Erythroxylon.

Wine of Coca.

Fluid Extract of Erythroxylon	1 fluidounce.
Alcohol	1 "
Sugar	1 troy ounce.
Claret Wine . . . . enough to make	16 fluidounces.

Dissolve the Sugar in about *ten* (10) *fluidounces* of Claret Wine, add the Alcohol and Fluid Extract, and enough Claret Wine to make *sixteen* (16) *fluidounces*. Let the mixture stand a few days in a cold place, if convenient, then filter and pass enough Claret Wine through the filter, to restore the original volume.

Each fluidounce represents 30 grains of Erythroxylon (Coca).

Note.—In place of Claret Wine, any other palatable wine may be used, according to the demand or preference of the prescriber or consumer.

430. VINUM ERYTHROXYLI AROMATICUM.

Aromatic Wine of Erythroxylon.

Aromatic Wine of Coca.

Fluid Extract of Erythroxylon	1 fluidounce.
Compound Elixir of Taraxacum	60 minims.
Syrup of Coffee	180 "
Port Wine	2½ fluidounces.
Aromatic Elixir	4½ "
Sherry Wine . . . . enough to make	16 "

Mix the five first-named ingredients with *seven* (7) *fluidounces* of Sherry Wine. Let the mixture stand several days in a cold place, if convenient, then filter, and pass enough Sherry Wine through the filter to make the product measure *sixteen* (16) *fluidounces*.

Each fluidounce represents 30 grains of Erythroxylon (Coca).

431. VINUM FRAXINI AMERICANÆ.

Wine of White Ash.

Fraxinus (bark) in No. 40 powder	8 troy ounces.
Stronger White Wine (U. S. P.) . . enough to make	16 fluidounces.

Moisten the powdered Fraxinus with *sixteen* (16) *fluidounces* of Stronger White Wine, macerate it during three days in a well covered vessel, then pack it in a percolator, and gradually pour on Stronger White Wine, until *sixteen* (16) *fluidounces* of percolate are obtained. Keep the product in well-stoppered bottles, which should be completely filled, and stored in a cool place.

Each fluidrachm represents 30 grains of Fraxinus (bark).

Note.—Fraxinus bark is the inner bark of the trunk or root of *Fraxinus Americana* Linné (White Ash).

432. VINUM PEPSINI.

Wine of Pepsin.

Pepsin (N. F.)	128 grains.
Glycerin	360 minims.
Hydrochloric Acid	30 "
Water	1 fluidounce.
Purified Talcum	120 grains.
Stronger White Wine (U. S. P.) . . . enough to make	16 fluidounces.

Mix the Water, Glycerin and Hydrochloric Acid, and agitate the Pepsin with the mixture until it is completely disintegrated and apparently dissolved. Then add enough Stronger White Wine to make *sixteen* (16) *fluidounces*, mix the liquid intimately with the Purified Talcum, allow it to stand for a week, if convenient, frequently shaking, then filter, and pass enough Stronger White Wine through the filter to restore the original volume.

Each fluidrachm represents 1 grain of Pepsin (N. F.).

433. VINUM PICIS.

Wine of Tar.

Tar	1½ troy ounces.
Water	4 fluidounces.
Pumice, in moderately fine powder	2 troy ounces.
Stronger White Wine . . . . enough to make	16 fluidounces.

Upon the Tar contained in a suitable vessel pour *four* (4) *fluidounces* of cold Water, and triturate the mixture thoroughly; then pour off the Water and throw it away. Mix the remaining Tar thoroughly with the powdered Pumice, and add *sixteen* (16) *fluidounces* of Stronger White Wine. Stir frequently during four hours, then transfer the mixture to a wetted filter, and, after the liquid has passed, pour on enough Stronger White Wine to make the filtrate measure *sixteen* (16) *fluidounces.*

434. VINUM PRUNI VIRGINIANÆ.

Wine of Wild Cherry.

Wild Cherry, in No. 40 powder	4 troy ounces.
Sugar	2½ " "
Water	3 fluidounces.
Alcohol	1 fluidounce.
Purified Talcum	120 grains.
Angelica Wine . . . . enough to make	16 fluidounces.

Dissolve the Sugar in the Water. Moisten the Wild Cherry with a sufficient quantity of this solution, and allow it to macerate during one hour. Then transfer it to a percolator, pour upon it the remainder of the solution, and afterwards, enough Angelica Wine until *fifteen* (15) *fluidounces* of percolate are obtained. Add to this the Alcohol, mix the Purified Talcum intimately with the liquid, then filter, returning the first portions of the filtrate until it runs through clear, and finally pass enough Angelica Wine through the filter, to make the product measure *sixteen* (16) *fluidounces.*

Each fluidrachm represents 15 grains of Wild Cherry.

435. VINUM PRUNI VIRGINIANÆ FERRATUM.

Ferrated Wine of Wild Cherry.

Tincture of Citro-Chloride of Iron		640 minims.
Wine of Wild Cherry	enough to make	16 fluidounces.

Mix the Tincture with enough Wine of Wild Cherry to make *sixteen* (16) *fluidounces.*

Each fluidrachm represents 5 minims of Tincture of Citro-Chloride of Iron and 13¾ *grains of Wild Cherry.*